ATLAS OF BIOPSY PATHOLOGY FOR HEART AND LUNG TRANSPLANTATION

ATLAS OF BIOPSY PATHOLOGY FOR HEART AND LUNG TRANSPLANTATION

Susan Stewart FRCPath

Consultant Respiratory Histopathologist,
Papworth Hospital NHS Trust, UK

Nathaniel R. B. Cary MD FRCPath

Consultant Cardiac Histopathologist,
Papworth Hospital NHS Trust, UK,
now Consultant Forensic Pathologist,
GKT School of Medicine, King's College,
Guy's Hospital, London, UK

Martin J. Goddard FRCS MRCPath

Consultant Cardiorespiratory Histopathologist,
Papworth Hospital NHS Trust, UK

Margaret E. Billingham MD FRCPath

Emerita Professor of Cardiac Pathology,
Stanford University, USA

A member of the Hodder Headline Group
LONDON
Co-published in the USA by Oxford University Press Inc., New York

First published in Great Britain in 2000 by
Arnold, a member of the Hodder Headline Group,
338 Euston Road, London NW1 3BH

http://www.arnoldpublishers.com

Co-published in the United States of America by
Oxford University Press Inc.,
198 Madison Avenue, New York, NY10016
Oxford is a registered trademark of Oxford University Press

Whilst the advice and information in this book are believed to be true and
accurate at the date of going to press, neither the authors nor the publisher
can accept any legal responsibility or liability for any errors or omissions
that may be made. In particular (but without limiting the generality of the
preceding disclaimer) every effort has been made to check drug dosages;
however it is still possible that errors have been missed. Furthermore,
dosage schedules are constantly being revised and new side-effects
recognized. For these reasons the reader is strongly urged to consult the
drug companies' printed instructions before administering any of the drugs
recommended in this book.

British Library Cataloguing in Publication Data
A catalogue record for this book is available from the British Library

Library of Congress Cataloging-in-Publication Data
A catalog record for this book is available from the Library of Congress

ISBN 0 340 69142 5

1 2 3 4 5 6 7 8 9 10

Commissioning Editor: Georgina Bentliff
Project Editor: Michael Lax
Production Editor: James Rabson
Production Controller: Fiona Byrne
Cover design: Julie Delf

Composition by Scribe Design, Gillingham, Kent, UK
Colour separation by Tenon & Polert Colour Scanning Ltd
Printed and bound in China

CONTENTS

Contents

FOREWORD

Transvenous endomyocardial biopsy was introduced by Philip Caves in 1974.[1] Until then the diagnosis of cardiac rejection was made largely on the basis of abnormal physical signs and declining ECG voltages. The latter used to be summated and charted twice daily during the early post-operative period. However, using these means, rejection was inevitably well advanced by the time it was detected, and consequently more difficult to reverse. Cardiac biopsy, relying as it did on the histological evidence of rejection before this had progressed to myocardial oedema and dysfunction, meant that treatment could be initiated earlier and also that there was better control over the duration for which augmented immunosuppression was necessary. Its introduction resulted in a marked improvement in outcome following cardiac transplantation, as evidenced by the Stanford experience, where, with no change in immunosuppressive protocol, the one-year survival improved from 45 to 60%.[2]

As a result of her work with cardiac biopsy, Margaret Billingham soon became the acknowledged world authority on the histological interpretation of rejection. Furthermore, any group contemplating heart transplantation soon recognised that access to accurate histopathology was essential for a successful programme. In the early days this often meant one or more visits to Stanford by the pathologist, so that he or she could learn from the experience already accumulated by Dr Billingham. Also, those responsible for the post-operative management of heart transplant patients had to have confidence in the accuracy of the biopsy reports they were receiving, and hence felt the need to be familiar with the histological appearances of rejection. How much easier it all would have been if this excellent Atlas of Pathology had been available to us twenty or even ten years ago!

The present text is a fitting culmination to the productive link that has existed between the pathologists at Stanford and Papworth for many years now and it deserves to be a great success. The Atlas is comprehensive, covering as it does not only the histology of rejection but also illustrating the salient histological features of infection and other pathology that is occasionally encountered in biopsy specimens of both heart and lung and ending with a useful appendix on handling and processing biopsies. The authors are also to be commended for the way in which the material is presented. The emphasis throughout is on the superb photomicrographs, supplemented by brief and accurate summaries that draw attention to the important histological appearances. In addition, an extensive and up to date list of references is conveniently provided at the end of each section.

I believe the authors have reason to be proud of all the hard work that must have gone into producing this Atlas, and that it will find a very appreciative audience, not only amongst professional pathology colleagues but also amongst all those who are responsible for managing the immunosuppression of heart and lung transplant patients.

Sir Terence English KBE, DL, FRCS

REFERENCES

1. Cave PK, Stinson EB, Billingham ME, Shumway NE. Percutaneous transvenous endomyocardial biopsy in human heart recipients (experience with a new technique). *Ann Thorac Surg* 1973; **16**: 325.
2. Griepp RB, Stinson EB, Bieber CP *et al.* Increasing patient survival following heart transplantation. *Transplant Proc* 1977; **9**: 197–201.

PREFACE

Cardiothoracic transplantation is an established therapy for end-stage heart and lung disease requiring specialist pathologic support. The histopathology of cardiac and pulmonary transplantation is now well described both in textbooks of pathology and clinical transplantation but these accounts are insufficient for the reporting pathologist supporting a cardiothoracic transplant program. We therefore decided to produce an *Atlas of Biopsy Pathology for Heart and Lung Transplantation* to address the need for a practical bench book. We have illustrated rejection, infection and other transplant pathologies with biopsies from two major international cardiothoracic centers where we have been involved in developing clinical transplantation and in the training of numerous visiting pathologists. We have emphasized the practical aspects of biopsy diagnosis with differentials and potential pitfalls given for each condition. Each section is introduced with brief text with the detail in the figures and legends. In this way we hope to have achieved a true Atlas rather than a lavishly illustrated textbook. Each section is extensively referenced for further reading. A background knowledge of cardiac and pulmonary pathology will be helpful but is not essential and we have included tables of key features to guide the specialist and non-specialist alike. The Atlas is also intended for transplant clinicians, including those in training, who need to appreciate the role of biopsies in monitoring treatment of the transplant recipient. The benefit of the multidisciplinary approach is emphasized throughout. We have not covered explant, cardiac or pulmonary pathology. The Atlas is in fact a companion book to *Practical Cardiovascular Pathology* by Sheppard and Davies which gives an up-to-date practical account of cardiac pathology.

The latest registry figures of the International Society of Heart Lung Transplantation show that there are 304 programs carrying out heart transplants, 124 heart–lung and 153 lung transplants world-wide. These have generated 48 541 heart recipients, 2510 heart–lung, 3751 double lung and 5347 single lung recipients illustrating the need for practical guidance for the reporting histopathologists in these centers. We have large referral practices and have supported transplant centers at a distance with biopsy services and anticipate that this Atlas will provide essential guidance in transplantation pathology.

We would like to acknowledge the support and encouragement of our clinical colleagues at Papworth and Stanford whose knowledge we have shared in establishing clinical heart and lung transplantation. We also acknowledge the technical excellence of our laboratory staff and the secretarial support from Miss Carolyn Hill in producing the manuscript.

Dr S Stewart
Dr NRB Cary
Dr MJ Goddard
Prof ME Billingham

PART 1

ENDOMYOCARDIAL BIOPSIES FOR HEART AND HEART–LUNG TRANSPLANT RECIPIENTS BASED ON INTERNATIONAL SOCIETY FOR HEART LUNG TRANSPLANTATION (ISHLT) GRADING SYSTEM

INTRODUCTION

Although many non-invasive methods have been tried, the endomyocardial biopsy remains the best method for monitoring a cardiac allograft for acute rejection. Several grading systems were established in different transplant centers in the early days of cardiac transplantation but a standard system, the International Society for Heart Lung Transplantation (ISHLT) grading system, was agreed in 1990 to standardize grading of rejection amongst pathologists for use both in publications and multicenter drug trials. The grading system requires adequacy of biopsy as well as standardization of a number of technical aspects of tissue examination. The various rejection grades are illustrated in Table 1 and additional information which should be included in the biopsy report is illustrated in Table 2.

There have in recent years, been attempts to modify and simplify the ISHLT grading system. The proposal was to include rejection grades from 1A, 1B and 2 in the 1990 grading system, in the modified Grade 1 whilst leaving the higher grades of rejection unchanged. However, there remains lack of uniformity in the management of Grade 2 rejection and most centers continue to use the 1990 grading system. The proposed modifications are also included in Table 1.

Table 2

Additional required information by ISHLT grading. Whilst the majority of endomyocardial biopsies will show varying grades of rejection, other features are not uncomonly seen and should be recorded. The key additional areas are listed in the table

Adequacy of biopsy	Adequate
	Inadequate tissue
	Inappropriate tissue
Evidence of infection	YES/NO
Organism identified	CMV
	Other
Endocardial infiltrate	With encroachment
	Without encroachment
Previous biopsy site	
Others	Peritransplant injury
	Myocardial vascular change
	Epicardial vascular change
	Epicardial inflammation
	Epicardial lipogranulomata
	Myocardial calcification
	Resolving/resolved rejection
	Ischemic/infarct damage

Table 1

Grading of cardiac rejection ISHLT (1990)

Old terms	Grades	Notes	Proposed simplification (1994)
No rejection	0	Biopsies with very sparse lymphoid infiltrates should be included in this grade	
'Mild' rejection	1A	Focal perivascular or interstitial infiltrates. The mild intensity and lack of myocyte damage distinguish this from higher grades	
	1B	Diffuse but sparse infiltrate. As with 1A, there must be no myocyte damage	Grade 1
'Focal' moderate rejection	2	One focus only with aggressive infiltration and/or focal myocyte damage. The choice of a single focus as the cut-off from higher grades is arbitrary. In practice, with the amount of tissue usually submitted, one is unlikely to be faced with the problem of biopsy fragments with only two foci	
Usual treatment threshold			
'Low' moderate rejection	3A	Multifocal aggressive infiltrates and/or myocyte damage. The multiple foci may be present in only one fragment or may be scattered throughout several fragments	Grade 3A
	3B	Diffuse inflammatory process. The intensity of the lymphoid infiltrate varies considerably. It may be little more than 1B, the important feature distinguishing it being the presence of myocyte damage. This damage must be present in at least two fragments, but some degree of infiltration is present in the majority of fragments	Grade 3B
'Severe acute' rejection	4	A diffuse and polymorphous infiltrate with or without edema, hemorrhage and vasculitis. The infiltrate is more intense and more widespread than 3B and myocyte damage is conspicuous. There are often neutrophils and/or hemorrhage, though neither is essential for diagnosis of this grade.	Grade 4

The grading system essentially grades rejection infiltrates in terms of both intensity and tendency to damage the myocardium. However it should always be borne in mind that whilst rejection is the commonest cause of mononuclear infiltrates post transplant, there are a number of other differential diagnoses to consider, in particular: – peritransplant injury, previous biopsy site, endocardial infiltrates, infection (*Toxoplasma gondii* and cytomegalovirus [CMV]) and lymphoproliferative disease.

Endomyocardial biopsy has become the established method of monitoring the graft as other clinical indices are less sensitive. Most centers biopsy according to protocols in the first 2 years post-transplant as clinically silent, but significant rejection occurs and has been associated with sudden death, presumably due to arrhythmia. Complications of the procedure are unusual.

The following sections illustrate the grades of rejection as well as the various other features which may be seen on endomyocardial biopsy post-transplant. Most endomyocardial biopsies are taken from heart transplant recipients but occasionally they will be performed on combined heart–lung recipients for the investigation of suspected cardiac abnormality. The histopathologic abnormalities are similar in both settings.

In order to make a diagnosis of acute rejection or to rule out acute rejection on a biopsy the ISHLT system requires there to be *at least four adequate pieces of tissue* and *six* if a smaller bioptome is used. An adequate piece of tissue is that which has more than 50% of evaluable myocardium (not adipose tissue or fibrosis or crush artefact). A size French 9 bioptome is preferred, but a size 7 French may be used. Bioptomes of 5–6 French (used for children) require a larger number of pieces of tissue to avoid sampling error.

In clinical practice, some information may be given on fewer fragments. If significant rejection is present in only three assessable fragments, then the presence of a fourth is immaterial. Similarly if three fragments show no evidence of infiltrate, then, the chance of missing significant rejection is small.

OTHER TECHNICAL CONSIDERATIONS

One or more additional endomyocardial biopsy fragments may be snap frozen for possible immunofluorescent studies/immunohistochemistry, though this is not mandatory. Formalin fixation and paraffin wax processing are standard. Sections should be cut from a minimum of three levels through the block and stained routinely with hematoxylin and eosin. H & E stained sections are usually adequate for the grading of the majority of biopsies. Additional stains such as Masson trichrome and elastic van Gieson stains can be of value in showing myocyte damage or fibrosis. Stains for organisms are also required on occasions as suggested either by clinical findings or histologic changes of necrosis, granulomas or unusual patterns of inflammation.

Box 1   Other considerations

Technical considerations
- Formalin fixation, paraffin processing
- Sectioning with minimum of three step levels

Requirements for grading
- Must have a minimum of four fragments at least 50% of each free from fibrosis or biopsy site
- To achieve this number reliably advise taking six or more fragments at a biopsy session

---

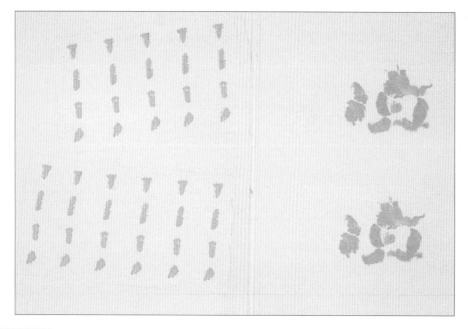

Figure 1.1
On the left-hand side an adequate biopsy set taken with a 9 French bioptome is illustrated with a biopsy set taken with a 7 French bioptome for comparison (right).

FURTHER READING

Alexis JD, Lao CD, Selter JG et al. Cardiac Troponin T : a non-invasive marker for heart transplant rejection? *J Heart Lung Transplant* 1998;**17**:395–8.

Billingham ME, Cary NRB, Hammond ME et al. A working formulation for the standardisation of nomenclature in the diagnosis of cardiac and lung rejection: heart rejection study group. *J Heart Transplant* 1990;**9**:587–93.

Billingham ME. The dilemma of variety of histopathological grading systems for acute allograft rejection by endomyocardial biopsy. *J Heart Transplant* 1990;**9**:272–6.

Blankenberg FG, Strauss HW. Non-invasive diagnosis of acute heart- or lung transplant rejection using radiolabeled annexin V. *Pediatr Radiol* 1999; **29**:299–305.

Cary NRB. Editorial: Grading of cardiac transplant rejection. *Heart* 1998;**79**:423–4.

Dengler TJ, Zimmermann R, Braun K et al. Elevated serum concentration of cardiac Troponin T in acute alllograft rejection after human heart transplantation. *J Am Coll Cardiol* 1998;**32**:405–12.

Fabregas RJ, Crespo-Leiro MG, Muniz J et al. Usefulness of pulsed Doppler tissue imaging for non-invasive detection of cardiac rejection after transplantation. *Transplant Proc* 1999;**31**:2545–7.

Hausen B, Albes JM, Rohden R, Demertzis S, Mugge A, Schafers HJ. Tricuspid valve regurgitation attributable to endomyocardial biopsies and rejection in heart transplantation. *Ann Thorac Surg* 1995; **59**:1134–40.

Moidl R, Chevtchik O, Simon P et al. Non-invasive monitoring of peak filling rate with acoustic quantification echocardiography accurately detects acute cardiac allograft rejection. *J Heart Lung Transplant* 1999;**18**:194–201.

Nakhleh RE, Bolman RM, Shumway S, Braulin E. Correlation of endomyocardial biopsy findings with electrocardiogram voltage in pediatric cardiac allografts. *Clin Transplant* 1992;**6**:114–8.

Nielsen H, Sorenen F, Nielsen B, Bagger JP, Thayssen P, Baandrup U. Reproducibility of the acute rejection diagnosis in human cardiac allografts: the Stanford classification and the international grading system. *J Heart Lung Transplant* 1993;**12**:239–43.

Pophal SG, Sigfusson G, Booth KL et al. Complications of endomyocardial biopsy in children. *J Am Coll Cardiol* 1999;**34**:2105–10.

Richantz BM, Radovancevic B, Bologna MT, Frazier OH. Usefulness of the QTc interval in predicting acute allograft rejection. *Thorac Cardiovasc Surg* 1998;**46**:217–21.

Rodriguiz ACAR, de Vylder A, Wellens F, Bartunek J, de Bruyne B. Right ventricular pseudoaneurysm as a complication of endomyocardial biopsy after heart transplantation. *Chest* 1995;**107**:566–7.

Roussoulieres AL, Schnetzler B et al. Haematoma of the interventricular septum following right ventricular endomyocardial biopsy for the detection of allograft rejection after heart transplantation. *J Heart Lung Transplant* 1999;**18**:1147–50.

Sethi GK, Kosarajo S, Arabia FA, Roasda LJ, McCarthy MS, Copeland JG. Is it necessary to perform surveillance endomyocardial biopsies in heart transplant recipients? *J Heart Lung Transplant* 1995;**14**:1047–51.

Stewart MJ, Huwez F, Richens D, Naik S, Wheatley DJ. Infective endocarditis of the tricuspid valve in an orthotopic heart transplant recipient. *J Heart Lung Transplant* 1996;**15**:646–9.

Stewart S, Cary NRB. The pathology of heart and lung transplantation. *Curr Diagnost Pathol* 1996;**3**:69–79.

Stobierska-Dzierzek B, Surdacki A, Frasik W et al. Evaluation of plasma cyclic GMP assay as a screening test for detection of acute cardiac allograft rejection. *J Heart Lung Transplant* 1998;**17**:969–71.

Suvarna SK, Kennedy A, Ciulli F, Locke TJ. Revision of the 1990 working formulation for cardiac allograft rejection: the Sheffield experience. *Heart* 1998;**79**:432–6.

Tugulea S, Ciubotaniu R, Colovai A et al. New strageties for early diagnosis of heart allograft rejection. *Transplantation* 1997;**64**:842–7.

Van Gelder T, Balk AH, Zondervan PE et al. C-reactive protein in the monitoring of acute rejection after heart transplantation. *Transplant Int* 1998;**11**:361–4.

Vasquez-Rodriguez JM, Crespo-Leiro MG, Pampin-Conde MF et al. Cardiac troponin-T is not a marker of biopsy proven cellular rejection. *J Heart Lung Transplant* 1999;**18**:172.

White JA, Guiraudon C, Pflugfelder PW, Kostuk WJ. Routine surveillance myocardial biopsies are unnecessary beyond one year after heart transplantation. *J Heart Transplant* 1995:**14**:1050–6

Williams MJ, Lee MY, DiSalvo TG et al. Biopsy induced flail tricuspid leaflet and tricuspid regurgitation following orthotopic cardiac transplantation. *Am J Cardiol* 1996;**77**:1339–44.

Winters GL, Marboe CC, Billingham ME. The International Society for Heart and Lung Transplantation grading system for heart transplant biopsy specimens: clarification and commentary. *J Heart Lung Transplant* 1998;**17**:754–60.

Winters GL, McManus BM. Consistencies and controversies in the application of the International Society for Heart and Lung Transplantation working formulation for Heart Transplant biopsy specimens. *J Heart Lung Transplant* 1996;**15**:728–35.

Winters GL. The challenge of endomyocardial biopsy interpretation in assessing cardiac allograft rejection. *Curr Opin in Cardiol* 1997;**12**:146–52.

GRADE 0 REJECTION

This grade denotes cardiac biopsies showing either no infiltrate or very minimal infiltrate. Infiltrates within intramyocardial or epicardial fat or scar tissue should not be scored. Swollen endothelial cells or interstitial cell nuclei should not be mistaken for infiltrating cells.

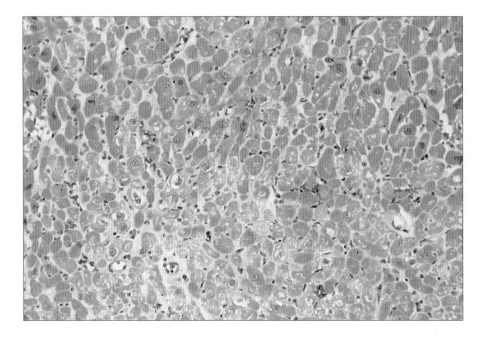

Figure 2.1
'Clean' biopsy entirely free of infiltrate.

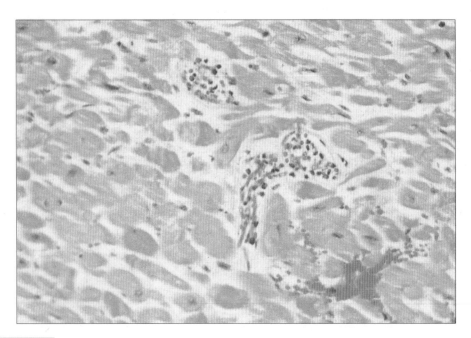

Figure 2.2
Biopsy showing cells mainly within small intramyocardial vessels should still be graded 0. The myocardium is free from infiltrating cells.

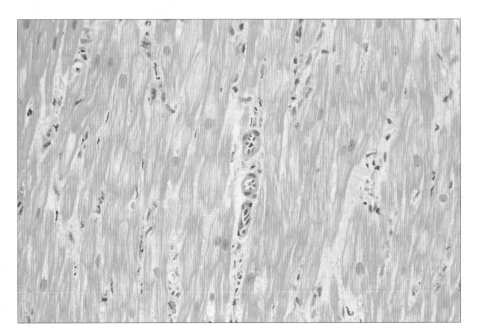

Figure 2.3
Swollen endothelial cell nuclei should not be confused with a rejection infiltrate. It is seldom if ever necessary to resort to immunohistochemistry to resolve this issue, as such minor infiltrates would be graded as 0 in any case.

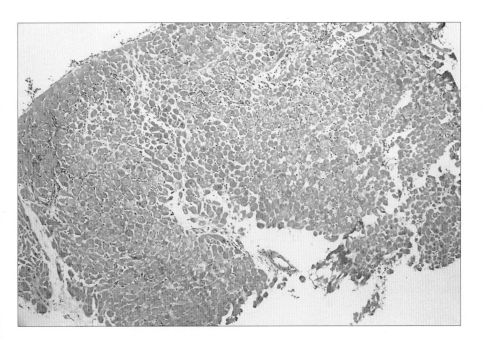

Figure 2.4
Biopsy showing scattered mononuclear infiltrates not associated with any myocyte damage. Biopsies where this is the maximum amount of infiltration present in all the serials are best graded as 0. The field illustrated is at the very upper limit of Grade 0.

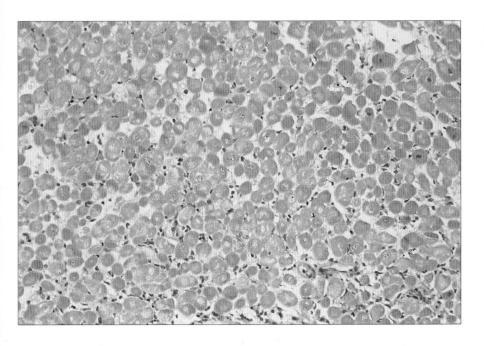

Figure 2.5
Higher magnification of the minimal infiltrate shown in 2.4.

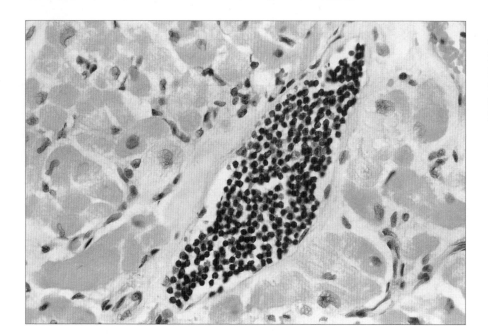

Figure 2.6
Occasionally vessels with the appearance of lymphatics and filled with mononuclear cells may be encountered. Biopsies showing this feature should also be included in Grade 0, providing of course there are no myocardial infiltrates present.

Box 2   Grade 0 rejection

- No infiltrate, or scattered very occasional mononuclear cells
- Differentiate from nuclei of swollen endothelial cells

FURTHER READING

Riseq MN, Masek MA, Billingham ME. Acute rejection: significance of lapsed time post transplant. *J Heart Lung Transplant* 1994;**13**:863–8.

Sharples LD, Cary NRB, Large SR, Wallwork J. Error rates with which endomyocardial biopsies are graded for rejection following cardiac transplantation. *Am J Cardiol* 1992;**70**:527–30.

Spiegelhalter DJ, Stovin PGI. An analysis of repeated biopsies following cardiac rejection. *Stats Med* 1983;**2**:33–40.

GRADES 1A AND 1B – MILD ACUTE REJECTION

GRADE 1A REJECTION

Focal predominantly perivascular or occasionally interstitial mononuclear infiltrates (lymphocytes, some macrophages and infrequent plasma cells) of mild intensity and not associated with myocyte encroachment or damage. In common with other solid organ grafts, the rejection infiltrates are perivascular.

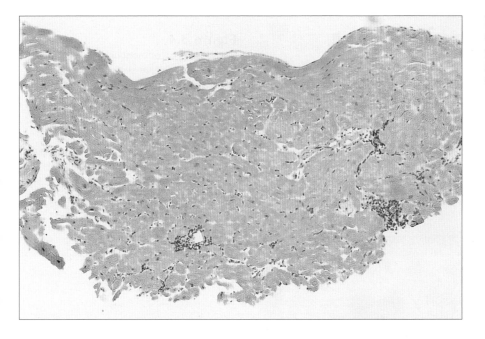

Figure 3.1
Grade 1A rejection. Three small areas of perivascular infiltration unassociated with myocyte damage. No evidence of endothelialitis is seen.

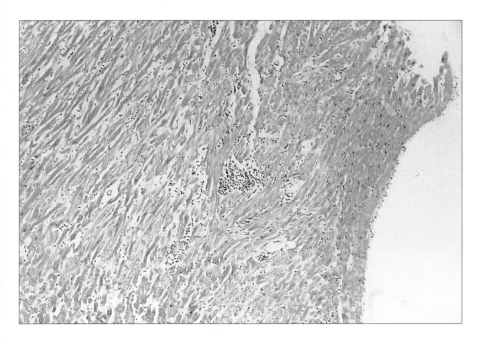

Figure 3.2
Low-power view showing a perivascular infiltrate of Grade 1A rejection.

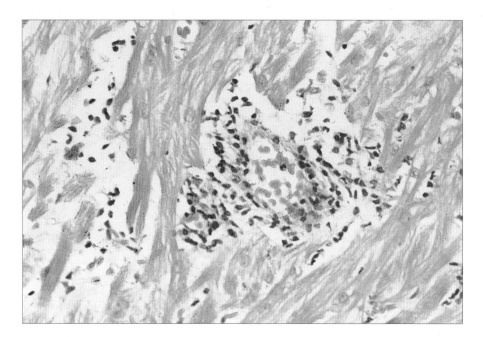

Figure 3.3
High-power view of the infiltrate in Fig. 3.2 showing its clear perivascular nature and its lack of any damage to adjacent myocytes.

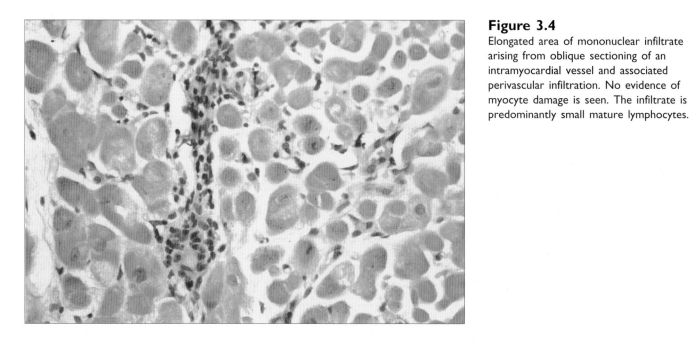

Figure 3.4
Elongated area of mononuclear infiltrate arising from oblique sectioning of an intramyocardial vessel and associated perivascular infiltration. No evidence of myocyte damage is seen. The infiltrate is predominantly small mature lymphocytes.

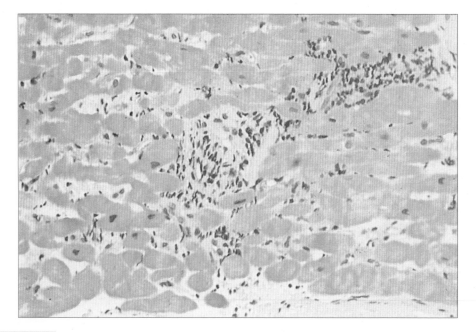

Figure 3.5
Although there is a conspicuous interstitial component to the mononuclear infiltrate present here, there is no convincing area of myocyte damage to suggest that this is moderate grade rejection. Deeper sections confirm the lack of myocyte damage.

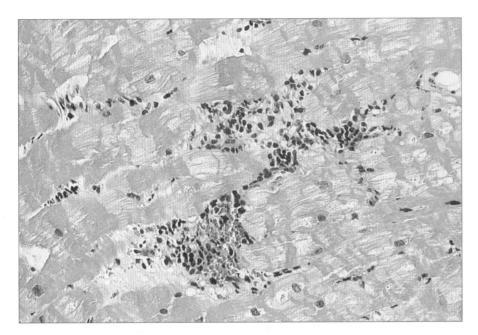

Figure 3.6
Both perivascular and interstitial infiltrates are present and in terms of the intensity this is towards the upper limit of that normally associated with Grade 1A. There is a suspicion of myocyte damage and on this field alone a definite decision could not be made as to whether this is simply 1A or in fact a focus of moderate rejection. Serial sections may resolve such an issue. Persistence of the infiltrate through numerous serials and/or evidence of myocyte damage would add weight to this being a focus of moderate rejection. If this were the case the biopsy would be given Grade 2, but would remain below the treatment threshold. Conspicuous contraction bands are seen in adjacent myocytes.

GRADE 1B REJECTION

Diffuse but sparse predominantly interstitial pattern of mononuclear infiltration. Although the process appears diffuse in medium- and high-power fields it is usually a focal process in terms of affecting only some areas of one or more of the biopsy fragments. There must be no evidence of myocyte damage. In practice this grade is rare compared with 1A. The differential diagnosis in Grade 1B is usually Grade 3B, where the infiltrate is more intense and widespread with clear evidence of myocyte damage.

Figure 3.7
Low-power view of the diffuse infiltrate characterizing 1B rejection.

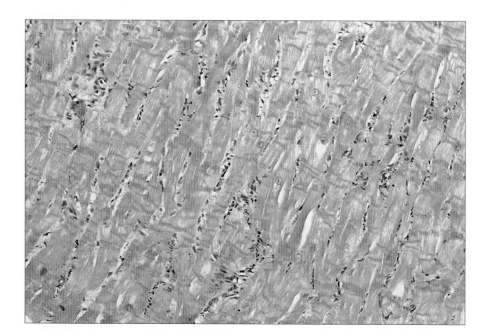

Figure 3.8
Low-power view of the diffuse infiltrate characterizing 1B rejection. Second fragment of same case as seen in Fig. 3.7.

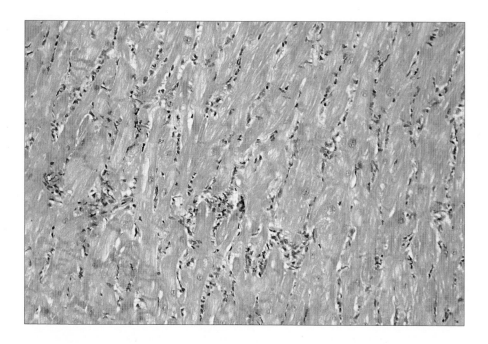

Figure 3.9
Low-power view of the diffuse infiltrate characterizing 1B rejection, slightly more intense than that shown in Figs 3.7 and 3.8, but nevertheless not obviously associated with myocyte damage in any area.

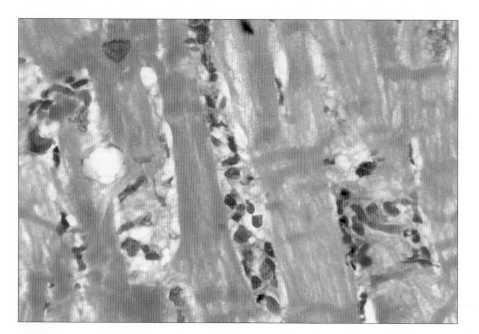

Figure 3.10
High-power view of Grade 1B rejection showing the mild nature of the infiltrate and its confinement to the interstitium without associated myocyte damage.

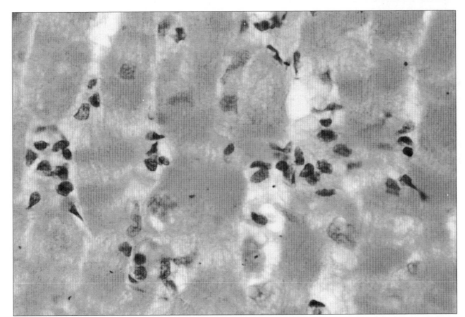

Figure 3.11
Further high-power view of Grade 1B rejection showing the mild nature of the infiltrate and its confinement to the interstitium without associated myocyte damage.

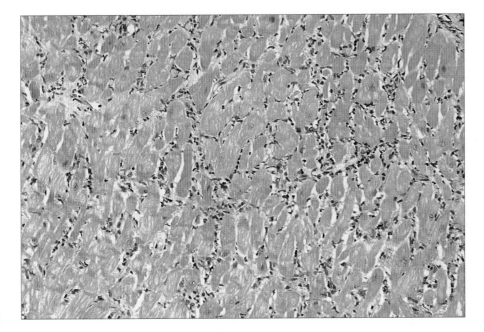

Figure 3.12
Difficult biopsy with diffuse infiltrate more intense than shown in the previous examples and with a suspicion of myocyte damage in some areas where myocytes are completely surrounded by infiltrating lymphocytes. Changes present in other fragments and the examination of multiple serials with usually resolve whether to grade as 1B or 3B.

Box 3   Grade 1A rejection

- One or more small foci of perivascular or interstitial mononuclear cells
- No evidence of myocyte damage in any of the foci of infiltration

---

Box 4   Grade 1B rejection

- Diffuse interstitial infiltrate of mononuclear cells of mild intensity and not associated with myocyte damage
- Amongst several fragments may nevertheless be a 'focal' process
- No difference in long-term follow-up between 1A and 1B

DEFINITION OF MODERATE ACUTE REJECTION

The term moderate acute rejection implies that the acute rejection process is causing myocyte damage. Increasing severity is defined by increasing numbers of inflammatory cells and increasing numbers of foci associated with increasing parenchymal and vascular damage. Difficulty arises in defining what histologic features constitute myocyte damage. Myocyte damage may appear as tinctorial or coagulative changes in the myocytes. However, damage is also implied by the infiltrate surrounding, or replacing the myocyte, producing irregular myocyte borders and architectural distortion. Lymphocytic nuclei may appear to lie within the myocyte. Furthermore, the lymphocytes appear enlarged and activated with oval or bean-shaped nuclei. The majority of cells are lymphoid but at higher grades eosinophils and neutrophils may also be seen.

There is a spectrum of myocyte damage from first one focus (Grade 2) to multiple foci (Grade 3A) and to diffuse infiltration in association with myocyte damage (Grades 3B and 4). Myocyte damage ranges from mononuclear infiltrate surrounding, scalloping and indenting the myocyte to frank necrosis of a myocyte or group of myocytes.

Box 5 Definition of moderate rejection

- Intensity of mononuclear infiltrate
- Evidence of myocyte damage
  - tendency of infiltrate to surround and replace myocytes
  - mononuclear cells encroaching on edges of myocyte cytoplasm
  - mononuclear cell nuclei within myocyte

Box 6 Nature of infiltrate in rejection grades

- Mononuclear infiltrate in rejection is a mixture of lymphocytes and macrophages
- Lymphocytes usually tend to be of larger type in higher grades of rejection, though not always
- Eosinophils are common though not invariable in higher grades of rejection
- Eosinophils may be seen in lower grades of rejection

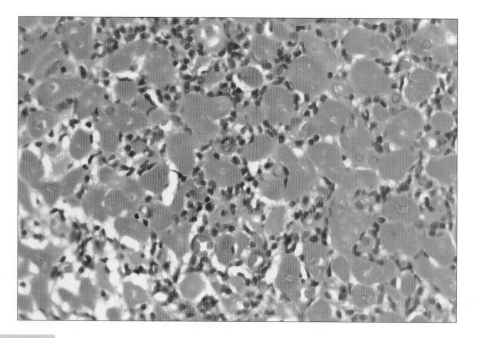

Figure 4.1
Focus of moderate rejection. The mononuclear infiltrate surrounds myocytes and in some areas has replaced them implying myocyte damage. Lymphocytes have enlarged and slightly irregular shaped nuclei.

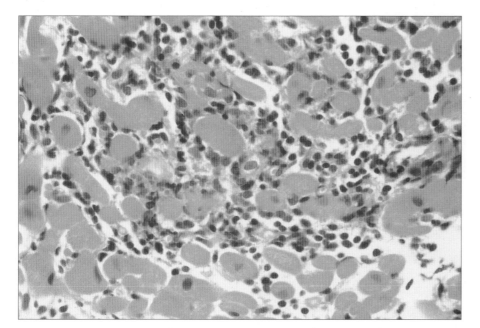

Figure 4.2
Focus of moderate rejection with more overt evidence of myocyte damage in terms of replacement by mononuclear infiltrate. There is obvious fragmentation and loss of integrity of the sarcoplasm with infiltrate seen within and impinging on several myocytes. Several individual myocytes are completely surrounded by infiltrate, a useful sign in less overt cases than this one.

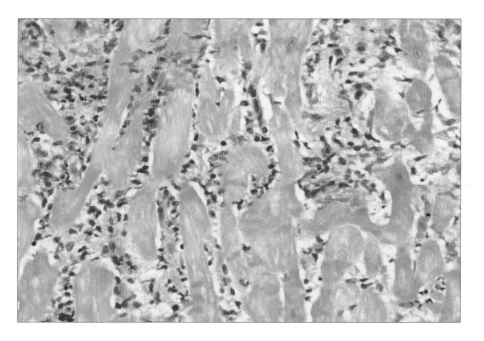

Figure 4.3
In diffuse moderate rejection (3B) the evidence of damage may be less obvious than in focal moderate rejection as is the case here. This grade is diagnosed on the basis both of intensity and diffuseness of infiltrate and the presence of myocyte damage in at least two fragments.

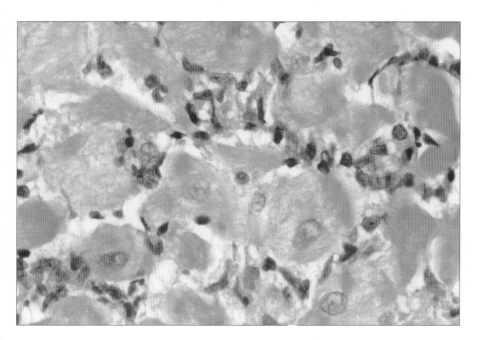

Figure 4.4
Myocyte damage in diffuse moderate rejection showing mononuclear infiltrates within sarcoplasm.

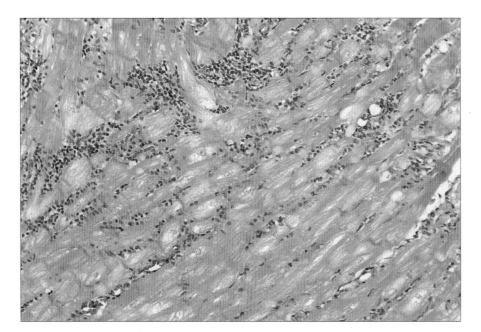

Figure 4.5

Moderate rejection, focal or diffuse?
Diagnostic difficulty can be encountered in deciding between 3A and 3B rejection. The other fragments are often of value. Presence of infiltrate even of a minor degree diffusely in all fragments will favor 3B whereas extensive 'clear' areas between 'foci' of moderate rejection will favor 3A. In practice, this makes no difference to treatment. Note the presence of eosinophils within the infiltrate.

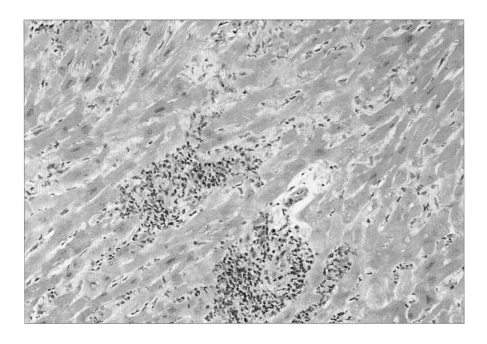

Figure 4.6

Two foci or one? A common sense approach should be adopted. The two adjoining foci illustrated here would probably be best viewed as one in grading terms. If these were the worst changes present then Grade 2 would be appropriate. If more widely separated by normal uninvolved myocardium they should be viewed as separate foci and graded as Grade 3A. The presence of eosinophils should also alert to the possibility of a higher grade, and in the symptomatic patient augmented immunosuppression advised.

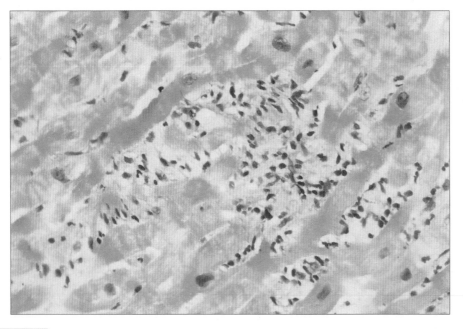

Figure 4.7 and 4.8

Small foci of infiltrate apparently associated with myocyte damage may on occasion cause difficulty either as the only change present in a biopsy set or as a finding in addition to one more obvious focus of moderate rejection. The former is relatively unimportant. However the latter will be relevant to the usual treatment threshold of 2 versus 3A. A case could be made either for upgrading or downgrading and there is clearly no obvious answer. Early on, peritransplant injury should always be considered for such changes and later on ischemia should be considered in the face of developing coronary disease. In Fig. 4.7 the presence of myocyte damage is clear, but in Fig. 4.8 the changes are more difficult to interpret, and would have to be viewed in the light of other changes present elsewhere.

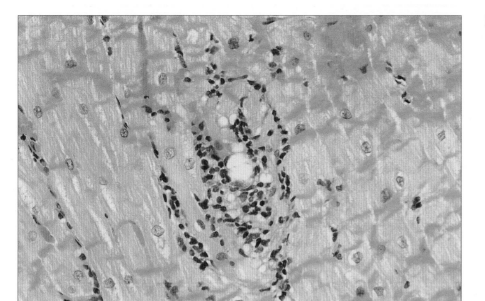

Figure 4.8

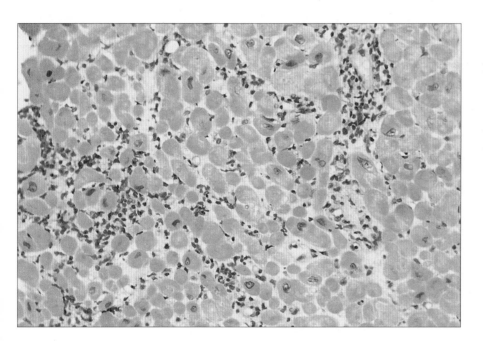

Figure 4.9
The infiltrate at the bottom right would be gradeable as mild. However that towards the top left lies at the border line of mild and moderate rejection. To some extent it is up to individuals to develop a consistent and preferably reproducible 'minimum' for the diagnosis of moderate rejection within an institution. In our institution, this would be gradeable as focus of moderate rejection (Grade 2) in a background of mild rejection.

FURTHER READING

Billingham ME, Cary NRB, Hammond ME *et al*. A working formulation for the standardisation of nomenclature in the diagnosis of cardiac and lung rejection : heart rejection study group. *J Heart Transplant* 1990;**9**:587–93.

di Gioia C R, d'Amati G, Grillo P, Lairenti A, Gallo P. Eosinophilic infiltration immediately following transplantation: recurrent hypersensitivity reaction? *Cardiovasc Pathol* 1999;**8**:297–9.

Dosanjh AK, Robinson TE, Strauss J, Berry G. Eosinophil activation in cardiac and pulmonary acute allograft rejection. *J Heart Lung Transplant* 1999;**17**:1038.

Myles JL, Ratliff NB, McMahon JT *et al*. Reversibility of myocyte injury in moderate and severe acute rejection in cyclosporin-treated cardiac transplant patients. *Arch Pathol Lab Med* 1987;**111**:947–52.

Stewart S, Cary NRB. The pathology of heart and lung transplantation. *Curr Diagnost Pathol* 1996; **3**:69–79.

Winters GL. The challenge of endomyocardial biopsy interpretation in assessing cardiac allograft rejection. *Curr Opin Cardiol* 1997;**12**:146–52.

GRADE 2 REJECTION

Grade 2 (focal rejection) is the most controversial grade of rejection for pathologists and clinicians. It is defined as a single focus fulfilling the criteria for moderate grade rejection in the whole biopsy set. No attempt is made in Grade 2 rejection to distinguish biopsies showing a single small focus from those showing a single large focus and no account is taken of whether or not other lesser grades of rejection co-exist. Careful studies using serial sections have demonstrated that many of these foci represent areas of encroaching endocardial infiltrate (*see*

Section 10). Furthermore, follow up studies on patients testify to the essentially benign nature of a Grade 2 biopsy, and that additional immunosuppression is not warranted. Some studies have suggested that a Grade 2 biopsy may be predictive of more significant rejection in the first 6 months; however protocol biopsies occur more frequently in this period and rejection is more common and thus the findings may not be fully indicative. The findings of Grade 2 in the first 6 months may warrant increased surveillance.

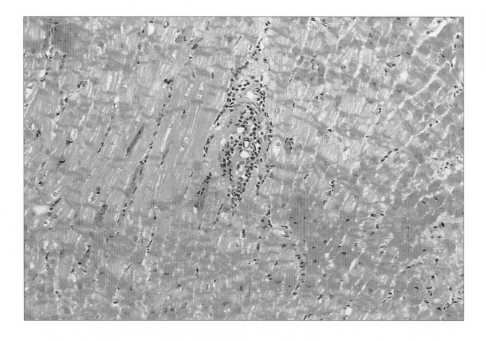

Figure 5.1
Low-power view showing single small focus of moderate rejection which was the only one in the whole biopsy set.

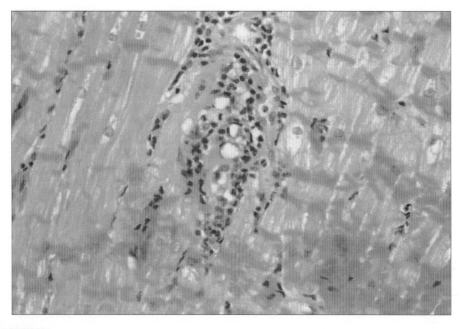

Figure 5.2
High-power view of a focus of moderate rejection showing that in spite of the small size of the focus there is undoubted evidence of myocyte damage.

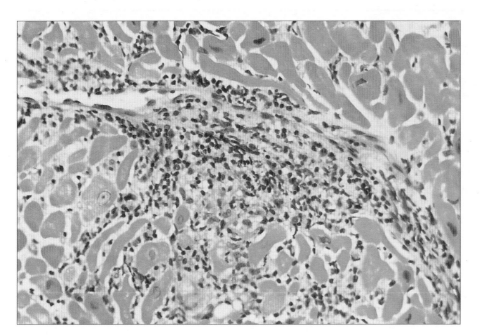

Figure 5.3
Large single focus of moderate rejection where the background showed evidence of IA rejection. If this were the only focus of moderate rejection it would still be graded as 2 as the highest numerical grade present in the biopsy determines the final grade. Note the presence of an endothelialitis with prominent endothelial cells in the vessels running across the section.

Box 7   Grade 2 rejection

- Single focus of moderate rejection amongst whole biopsy set
- May or may not be in a background of mild rejection
- Benign native Grade 2 established
- Many apparent foci of moderate rejection. May be encroaching endocardial infiltrate

---

FURTHER READING

Brunner-La Rocca HP, Sutsch G, Schneider J, Follath F, Kiowski W. Natural course of moderate cardiac allograft rejection (International Society for Heart transplantation grade 2) early and late after transplantation. *Circulation* 1996;**94**:1334–38.

El Gamel A, Doran H, Aziz T *et al*. Natural history and the clinical importance of early and late Grade 2 cellular rejection following cardiac transplantation. *Trans Proc* 1998;**30**:1143–6.

El Gamel A, Doran H, Rahman D, Deiraniya A, Campbell C, Yonan N. Clinical importance of grade 2 cellular heart rejection. *J Heart Lung Transplant* 1996;**15**:319–21.

Fishbein MC, Bell G, Lones MA *et al*. Grade 2 cellular heart rejection: does it exist? *J Heart Lung Transplant* 1994;**13**:1051–57.

Forbes RD, Rowan RA, Billingham ME. Endocardial infiltrates in human heart transplants: a serial biopsy analysis comparing full immunosuppression protocols. *Human Pathol* 1990;**21**:850–5.

Joshi A, Masek MA, Brown BW, Weiss LM, Billingham ME. Quilty revisited: a 10 year perspective. *Human Pathol* 1994;**26**:547–57.

Kemnitz J. Grade 2 Cellular heart rejection: does it exist?: Yes! *J Heart Lung Transplant* 1995;**14**:800–1.

Milano A, Caforio ALP, Livi U *et al*. Evolution of focal moderate (International Society for Heart transplantation grade 2) rejection of the cardiac allograft. *J Heart Lung Transplant* 1996;**15**:458–60.

Pardo-Mindan FJ and Lozano MD. 'Quilty effect' in heart transplantation: is it related to acute rejection? *J Heart Lung Transplant* 1991;**10**:937–41.

Winters GL, Loh E, Schoen F. Natural history of focal moderate cardiac allograft rejection. Is treatment warranted? *Circulation* 1995;**91**:1975–80.

GRADE 3A REJECTION

Two or more foci fulfilling the criteria of moderate rejection either seen within the same fragment or scattered amongst the biopsy fragments. However, each of the foci must independently fulfil the criteria for moderate rejection as discussed in Section 4. Most of the intervening myocardium is 'clean' in this grade. There may of course be other foci of mild rejection. The major differential is toxoplasma myocarditis, where the infiltrate may have more plasma cells and cysts are seen.

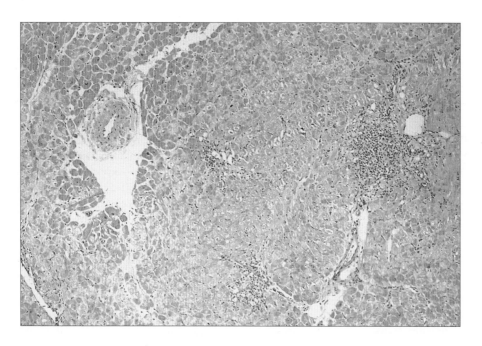

Figure 6.1
Three foci of moderate rejection which fortuitously for the purpose of illustration happen to all be visible within the same low-power field. More usually the two or more foci fulfilling the criteria of moderate rejection are scattered throughout the biopsy set either in different fragments and/or at different levels.

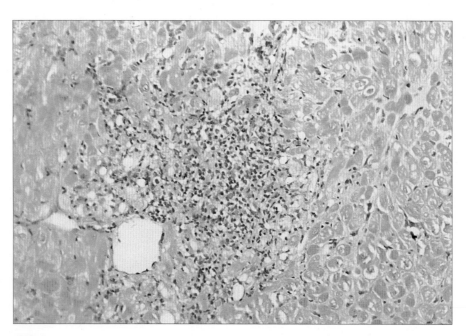

Figure 6.2
Intermediate power of the largest focus of moderate rejection seen in Fig. 6.1 illustrating the extent of the mononuclear infiltrate and its tendency to replace myocytes.

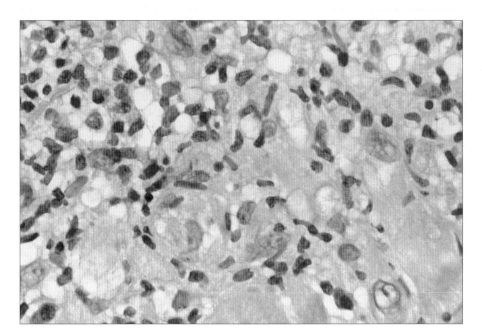

Figure 6.3
High-power view of an area of Fig. 6.2 showing evidence of on-going myocyte damage and replacement by infiltrate characterizing moderate rejection. Note enlarged lymphocytes within myocyte sarcoplasm.

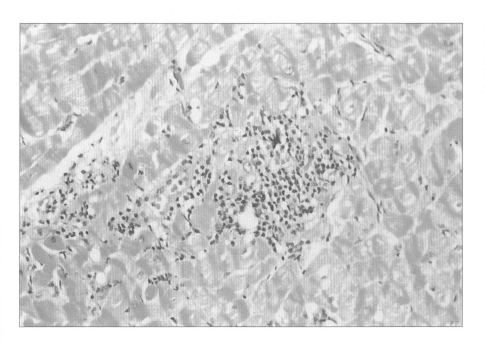

Figure 6.4
Discrete focus of moderate rejection. Note surrounding uninvolved myocardium with no infiltrate. Similar foci were present in other fragments to make this Grade 3A.

Box 8 Grade 3A rejection

* Multiple (i.e. two or more) foci of moderate rejection amongst whole biopsy set
* Foci may all be confined to one fragment or may be spread amongst several

Diffuse mononuclear infiltrates associated with myocyte damage in at least two biopsy fragments. Early after transplantation, this grade may be confused with peritransplant injury where there is myocyte damage and a diffuse infiltrate, although the infiltrate usually contains more macrophages and polymorphs in the latter.

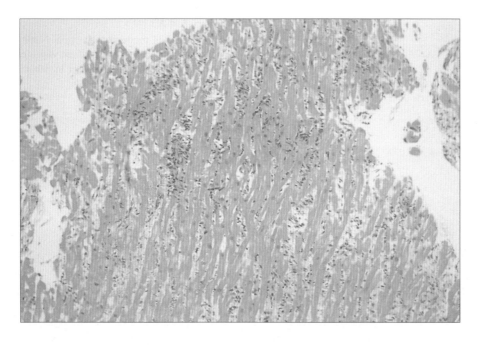

Figure 7.1
Grade 3B rejection, low-power. Compared with 3A, the infiltrate is more diffuse. Whilst there may be more intense foci of infiltration the intervening myocardium is also extensively infiltrated and myocyte damage is widespread. These changes were present in all fragments. Although the minimum requirement is at least two of the fragments, in most cases this is exceeded with little normal myocardium.

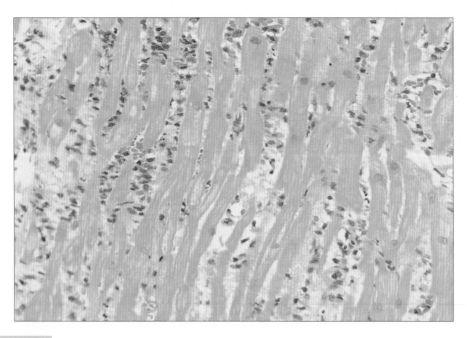

Figure 7.2
3B rejection, intermediate power illustrating the diffuseness of the infiltrate compared with 3A. The intensity of the infiltrate and the presence of myocyte damage both distinguish this from 1B.

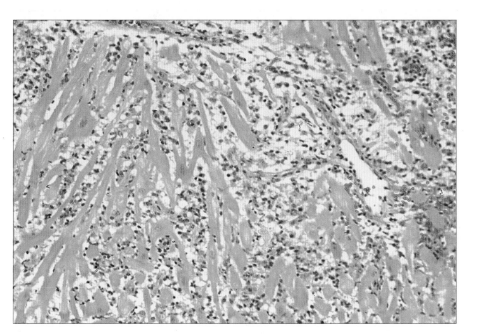

Figure 7.3
More florid diffuse infiltrate with some eosinophils, neutrophils and edema. This is towards the upper limit of Grade 3B.

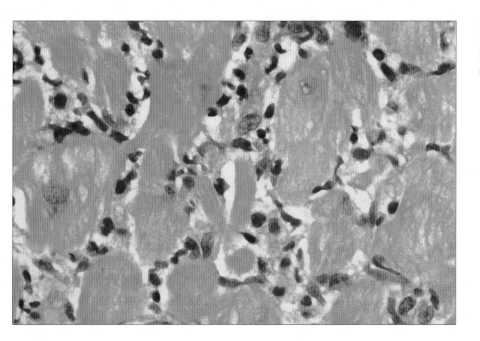

Figure 7.4
High-power view illustrates the diffuse infiltrate between all myocytes with conspicuous myocyte damage.

Box 9   Grade 3B rejection

- Diffuse mononuclear infiltrate in the majority of fragments associated with myocyte damage in at least two

GRADE 4 REJECTION

A diffuse infiltrate present in all fragments and associated with widespread damage and conspicuous edema. Hemorrhage is common but not essential to diagnose this grade. Some neutrophils are almost always present. This grade is very rare on cyclosporine-based immuno-suppression, but may be seen if medication is discontinued for any reason. There is a continuum from the changes of Grade 3B and in current practice the highest grade ever likely to be seen lies at the borderline of 3B and 4.

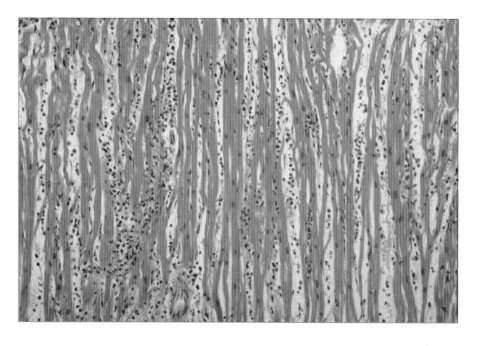

Figure 8.1
Grade 4 rejection. Note the diffuse nature of the infiltrate and the conspicuous edema leading to an appearance of widely separated myocytes. When this latter change is as florid as this there is no difficulty in diagnosing edema. However caution should be exercised when changes are rather less than this as artefacts arising from necessary rapid processing are common. The cellular infiltrate is typically mixed with neutrophils and eosinophils.

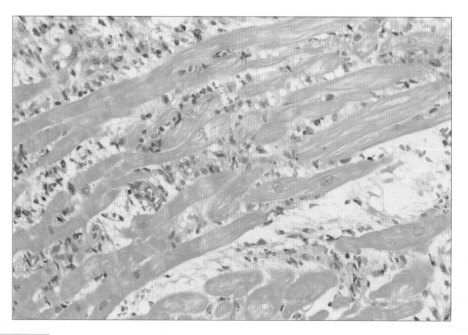

Figure 8.2
Areas from a case of Grade 4 rejection showing widespread edema and focal red cell extravasation. There is myocyte damage.

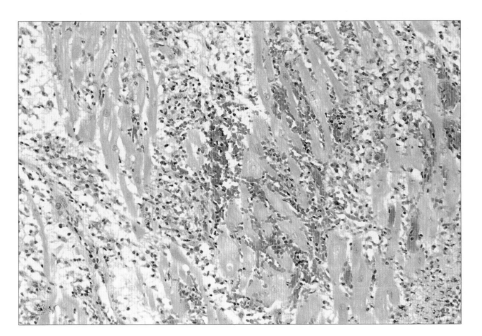

Figure 8.3
Intermediate-power of the hemorrhage and edema. Hemorrhage is a common biopsy artefact. However the extent and the context in which it is present make it likely to be genuine in this case.

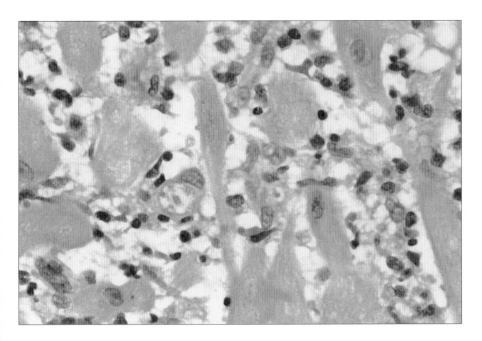

Figure 8.4
High-power of edema shown in Fig. 8.2. Note association with a mixed infiltrate with obvious myocyte damage seen as fragmentation and 'melting away' of cytoplasm.

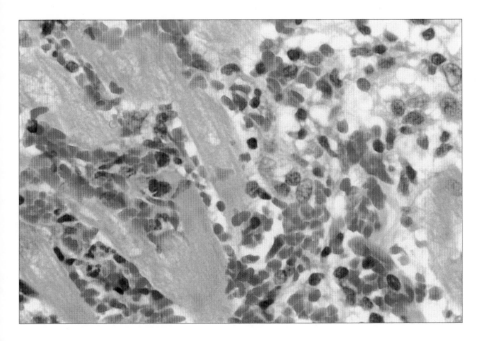

Figure 8.5
High-power of hemorrhage shown in Fig. 8.2. Hemorrhage results from complete disruption of capillary walls in association with infiltrate and obvious myocyte damage.

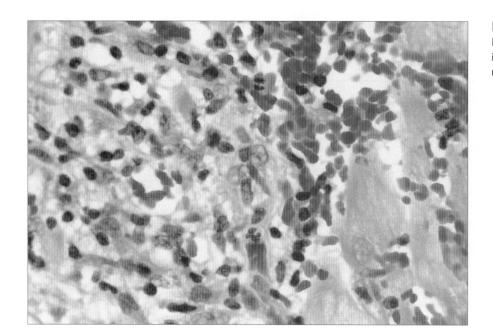

Figure 8.6
High-power of infiltrate shown in Fig. 8.2 illustrating the presence of a few neutrophils.

Box 10   Grade 4 rejection

- Diffuse infiltrate present in all fragments and associated with widespread myocyte damage
- Infiltrate more polymorphous than in other grades
- Eosinophils, neutrophils, hemorrhage and edema all common though none is essential for diagnosing this grade

RESOLVING AND RESOLVED ACUTE REJECTION

RESOLVING ACUTE REJECTION

If a subsequent or follow-up biopsy is diagnosed with a *lesser* grade than the previous biopsy, usually following treatment, then the biopsy can also be termed *resolving* in parenthesis following the numerical grade.

There is no absolute way of confidently diagnosing resolution in terms of positive features on biopsy. On occasion features such as a 'healing' infiltrate of mainly fibroblasts and macrophages with fewer residual small (inactive lymphocytes) and early fibrosis may be seen on biopsies taken as a follow up to rejection.

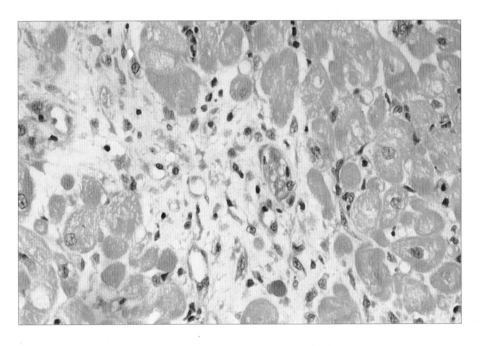

Figure 9.1
Follow-up biopsy to an episode of 3A rejection showing a focus of myocyte loss associated with a sparse mononuclear infiltrate. This could well represent the resolution of a previous focus of moderate rejection. Note the presence of some pigmented macrophages.

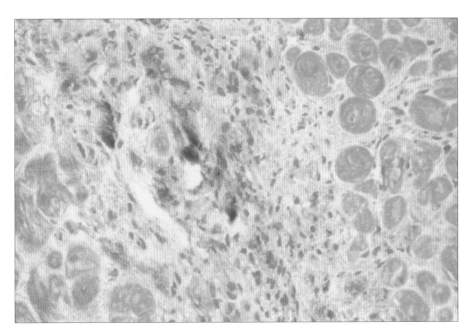

Figure 9.2
Hemosiderin deposits (blue) are seen in this area of presumed rejection related damage where some infiltrate still persists. (Perls' Prussian blue reaction). The presence of iron is neither specific for, nor diagnostic of a focus of resolving rejection.

RESOLVED ACUTE REJECTION

This term can be used if a biopsy shows no evidence of inflammatory infiltrate but only scar tissue following a previous recent (within 2 weeks) biopsy with a Grade 2 or higher. The biopsy can be Graded 0 with the word 'resolved' in parenthesis following the numerical grade.

Box 11   Other features to note
• Biopsy site
• Fibrosis
• Endocardial infiltrates
• Peritransplant (ischemic) injury
• Lymphoproliferative disease
• Infection (therefore ungradeable for rejection)
• Other

ENDOCARDIAL INFILTRATION

Prominent endocardial infiltrates or 'Quilty effect' as termed by Margaret Billingham are not an uncommon finding in the cyclosporine era of immunosuppression. They are foci of mononuclear cell infiltrate, which may have a prominent plasma cell population. Blood vessels with a prominent endothelial lining are typically found within them. They may be confined to the endocardium (Quilty A) or encroach on the underlying myocardium (Quilty B) even showing evidence of myocyte damage.

The cells include T-cells and macrophages but they also have a significant population of B cells. There has been no demonstrated difference in outcome between Quilty A and B lesions.

The etiology is unclear but the association with cyclosporine is well-established and mechanisms including a drug-specific effect, drug-related endothelial injury, and reduced endocardial drug levels are postulated.

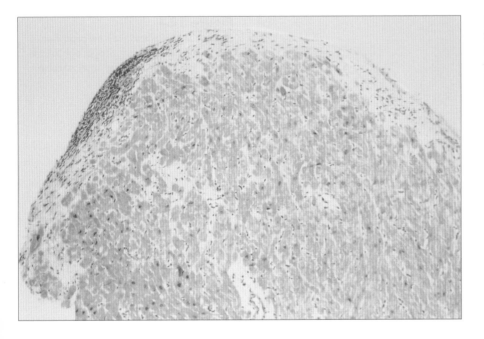

Figure 10.1
Small focus of non-encroaching endocardial infiltrate. Such foci are common in post-transplant endomyocardial biopsies. Underlying myocardium is free from infiltrate.

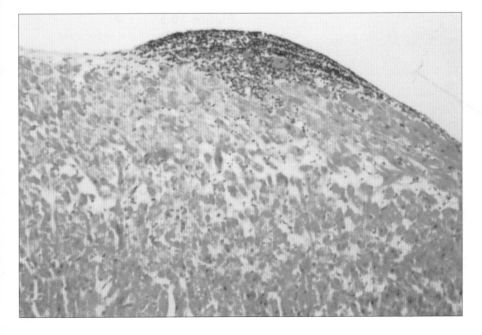

Figure 10.2
Endocardial infiltration with superficial encroachment, the so-called Quilty effect. Again this is common post-transplant and may be seen with or without rejection of the deeper myocardium. In this case, underlying myocardium is free of infiltrate.

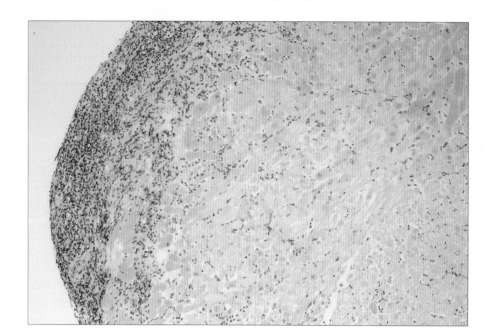

Figure 10.3
A more florid endocardial infiltrate involving the underlying myocardium with a suspicion of myocyte damage which should not be interpreted as rejection.

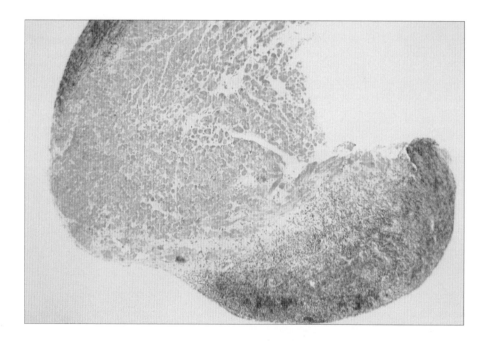

Figure 10.4
Endocardial infiltrates may be prominent and occupy a significant proportion of the biopsy. Even at low-power, the vascular pattern can be appreciated.

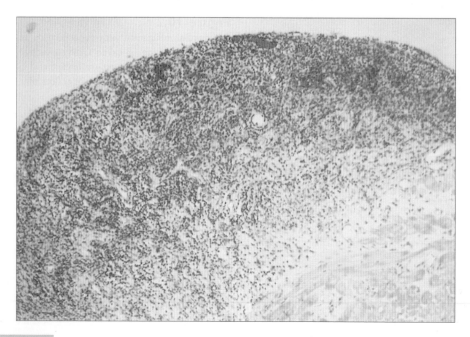

Figure 10.5
High-power view of the endocardial infiltrate. The infiltrate appears denser than normally seen in rejection and vessels are lined by prominent endothelial cells.

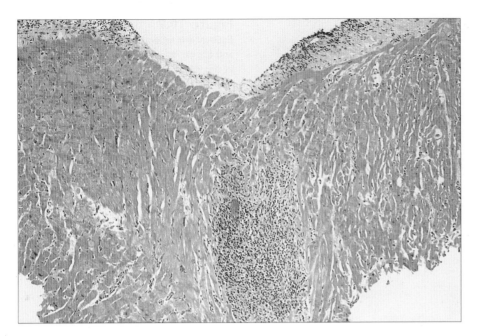

Figure 10.6
There is an infiltrate associated with myocyte damage, apparently present in deep myocardium.

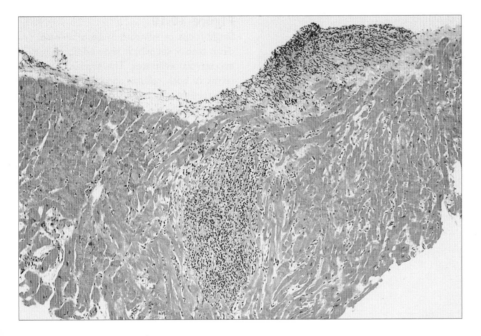

Figure 10.7 and 10.8
Deeper (or more superficial) sections clarify the true endocardial nature of this infiltrate which is due to both encroachment and tangential cutting make it appear to be in deep myocardium in Fig. 10.6. Such appearances may be mistaken for a focus of moderate rejection. However appreciation of this phenomenon together with an assessment of the nature and architecture of the infiltrate usually allow one to be suspicious of this as endocardial infiltration, even in the absence of being able to demonstrate a surface connection in other sections. This emphasizes the importance of serial sections.

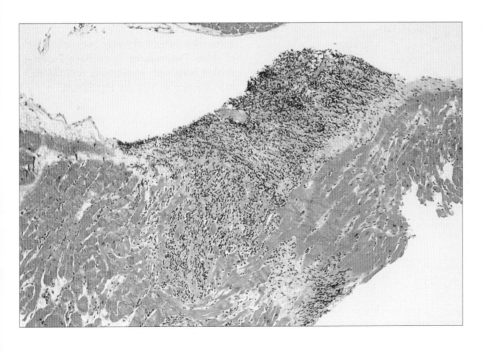

Figure 10.8

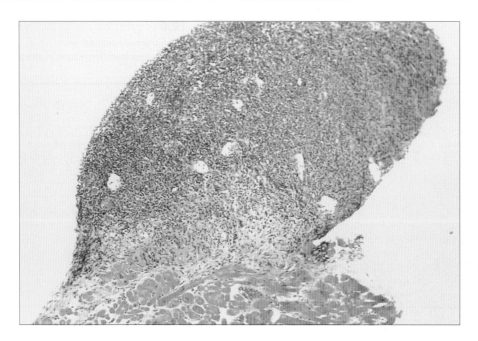

Figure 10.9
Endocardial infiltrate may appear very florid and appear as nodular lymphoid masses as in this case. The extent of these masses may be exaggerated by tangential cutting. The small and regular appearance of the infiltrate separates these from post-transplant lymphoproliferative disorder (PTLPD).

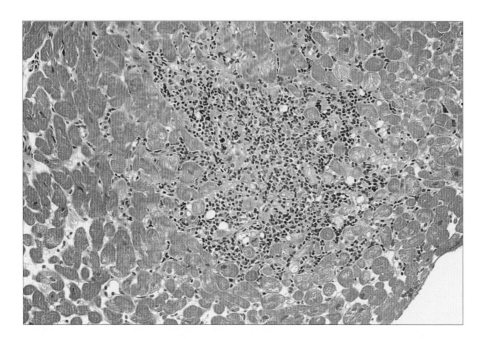

Figure 10.10
Single focus of infiltrate in an otherwise clean biopsy set which showed florid endocardial infiltrates. The similarity in terms of both cellular composition and architecture suggested that this was a focus of tangentially cut endocardial infiltrate even though no surface connection was demonstrated. A cautious approach is advisable, however, and when in doubt absence of any surface connection to a focus of myocardial infiltrate associated with damage should lead to a diagnosis of one (or more) foci of moderate rejection.

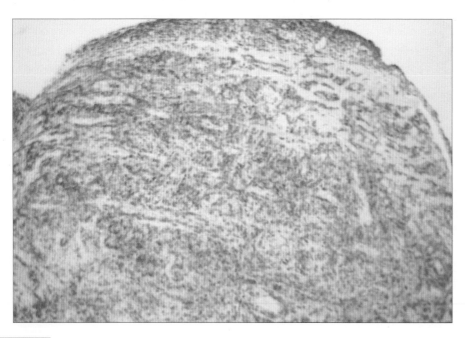

Figure 10.11
Immunohistochemistry may occasionally be of value. The majority of cells are T-cells stained here with an antibody to CD45RO. Non-staining vessels are highlighted.

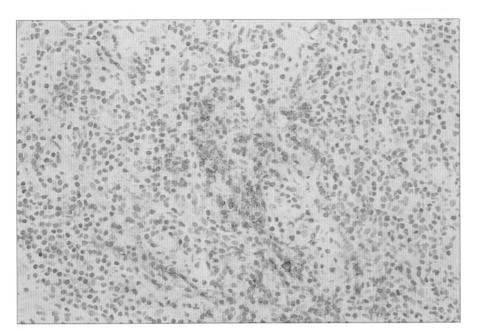

Figure 10.12
Groups of B-cells here stained with antibody to CD20 are usually present.

Box 12 Endocardial infiltrates

- Mixture of cells
- Vascularity may be prominent
- No difference in long-term follow-up between encroaching and non-encroaching infiltrates

---

FURTHER READING

Costanzo-Nordin MR, Winters GL, Fisher SAG *et al.* Endocardial infiltrates in the transplanted heart: clinical significance emerging from the analysis of 5026 endomyocardial biopsy specimens. *J Heart Lung Transplant* 1993;**12**:741–7.

Forbes RD, Rowan RA, Billingham ME. Endocardial infiltrates in human heart transplants: a serial biopsy analysis comparing full immunosuppression protocols. *Human Pathol* 1990;**21**:850–5.

Freimark D, Czer L, Aleksic I *et al.* Pathogenesis of Quilty lesion in cardiac allografts: relationship to reduced endocardial cyclosporine. *J Heart Lung Transplant* 1995;**14**:1197–1203.

Gopal S, Narasimhan U, Day JD *et al.* The Quilty lesion enigma: focal apoptosis/necrosis around lymphocyte subsets in human cardiac allografts. *Pathol Int* 1998;**48**:191–8.

Joshi A, Masek MA, Brown BW, Weiss LM, Billingham ME. Quilty revisited: a 10 year perspective. *Human Pathol* 1994;**26**:547–57.

Joshi A. The Quilty effect: current knowledge and clinical implications. *Trans Proc* 1998;**30**:907–8.

Kottke-Marchant K, Ratliff NB. Endomyocardial lymphocytic infiltrates in cardiac transplant recipients. *Arch Pathol Lab Med* 1989;**113**:690–8.

Pardo-Mindan F J and Lozano M D. 'Quilty effect' in heart transplantation: is it related to acute rejection? *J Heart Lung Transplant* 1991;**10**:937–941.

Radio SJ, McManus BM, Winters GL *et al.* Preferential endocardial residence of B-cells in the 'Quilty effect' of human heart allografts: Immunohistochemical distinction from rejection. *Mod Pathol* 1991;**4**:654–60.

Suit PF, Kottke-Marchant K, Ratliff NB, Pippenger C, Easely K. Comparison of whole blood cyclosporine levels and the frequency of endomyocardial lymphocytic infiltrates (the Quilty lesion) in cardiac transplantation. *Transplantation* 1989;**48**:618–21.

Small focal areas of myocyte damage may result from endogenous catecholamine-related damage in the donor prior to organ harvest, organ preservation and reperfusion or exogenous catecholamines given following implantation. This feature is common in early biopsies post-transplant. Cellular infiltrates may accompany peritransplant injury during resolution and must be distinguished from rejection. The infiltrate is usually mixed with polymorphs and macrophages, but lymphocytes and plasma cells may also be present. Lymphocytes may become more prominent later, but usually the infiltrate is within interstitium and perivascular spaces and not encroaching on viable myocytes. Concurrent ischemic injury and rejection may occur and can cause diagnostic difficulty. Ischemic injury has been identified as a risk factor for the development of graft vasculopathy in transplant patients.

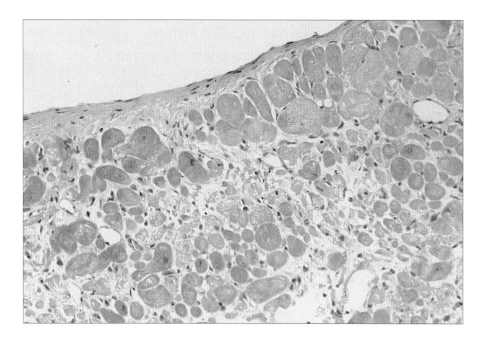

Figure 11.1
Peritransplant injury, low-power. Small foci of myocyte damage, often sub-endocardially, characterize this lesion. Myocytes are degenerate and poorly defined with no significant associated infiltrate.

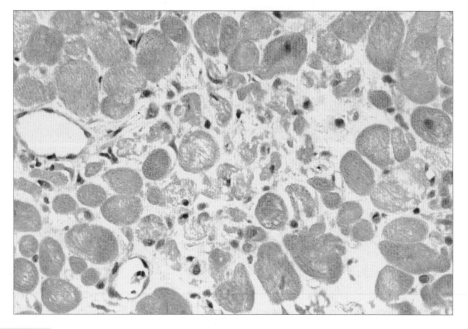

Figure 11.2
Peritransplant injury, high-power. Damaged myocytes appear to be 'melting away' without any inflammatory reaction at this stage. Such features are readily distinguished from rejection. Even at a later stage when cellular infiltration may occur it is usually possible to discriminate this from rejection as the degree of myocyte damage is disproportionate to the amount of infiltrate. Difficulties however may arise when recent enhanced immunosuppression has been given as this could lessen the degree of rejection associated infiltration. Knowledge of the time post-transplant and recent enhanced immunosuppression may be helpful in assessing the biopsy.

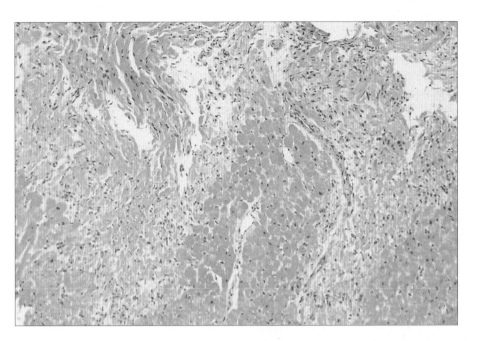

Figure 11.3
Low-power. Some early biopsies post-transplant may show particularly florid changes such as those present here where there are large areas of myocyte damage. Such changes are particularly liable to be seen in hearts which have had a long ischemic time, though not necessarily so.

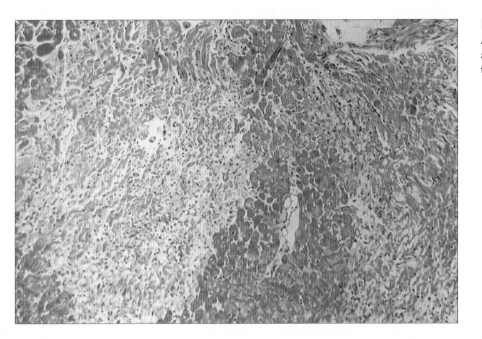

Figure 11.4
Areas of myocyte loss are much more apparent in this trichrome stained section from the same case as Fig. 11.3.

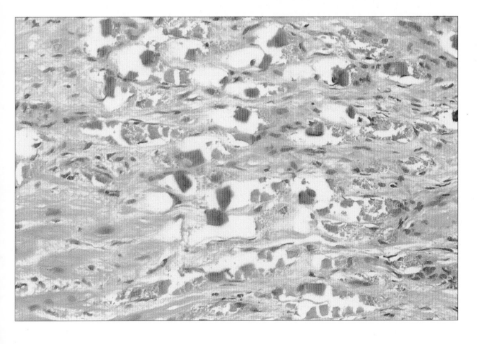

Figure 11.5
Old ischemic damage may be marked by dystrophic calcification of myocytes.

FURTHER READING

Baldwin WH, Samaniego-Picota M, Kasper EK *et al.* Complement deposition in early cardiac transplant biopsies is associated with ischaemic injury and subsequent rejection episodes. *Transplantation* 1999;**68**:894–900.

Davis SF, Yeung AC, Meredith IT *et al.* Early endothelial dysfunction predicts the development of transplant coronary artery disease at 1 year post transplant. *Circulation* 1996;**93**:457–62.

Day JD, Rayburn BK, Gaudin PB *et al.* Cardiac allograft vasculopathy; the central pathogenic role of ischaemic induced endothelial cell injury. *J Heart Lung Transplant* 1995;**14**:5142–9.

Fyfe B, Loh E, Winters GL, Couper G, Kartashov A, Schoen F. Heart transplantation-associated peri-operative ischaemic myocardial injury. Morphological features and clinical significance. *Circulation* 1996; **93**:1133–40.

Gaudin PB, Rayburn BK, Hutchins GM *et al.* Peritransplant injury to the myocardium associated with the development of accelerated arteriosclerosis in heart transplant recipients. *Am J Surg Pathol* 1994;**18**:338–46.

Labarrere CA, Nelson DR, Faulk WP. Myocardial fibrin deposits in the first month after transplantation predict subsequent coronary artery disease and graft failure in cardiac allograft recipients. *Am J Med* 1998;**105**:207–13.

Panizo A, Pardo F J, Lozano MD, de Alava E, Sla I, Idoate MA. Ischaemic injury in post-transplant endomyocardial biopsies : immunohistochemical study of fibronectin. *Trans Proc* 1999;**31**:2550–1.

Possible infective causes of infiltrates in post-transplant endomyocardial biopsies should always be considered, though in practice they are rare. Inflammatory infiltrates may be mixed, for instance including plasma cells, there may be evidence of acute inflammation with neutrophils or inflammation may be obviously granulomatous.

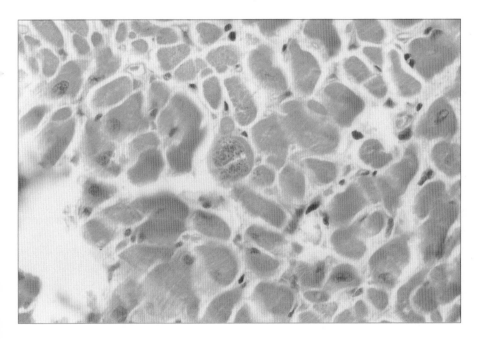

Figure 12.1
Endomyocardial biopsy showing cyst of *Toxoplasma gondii* within the myocyte cytoplasm. Note the lack of inflammatory infiltrate which if present may be in areas where no cysts are recognized, but may be due to extrusion of trophozooites. Fortunately toxoplasma is very rare now, due to pyremethamine or co-trimxazole prophylaxis.

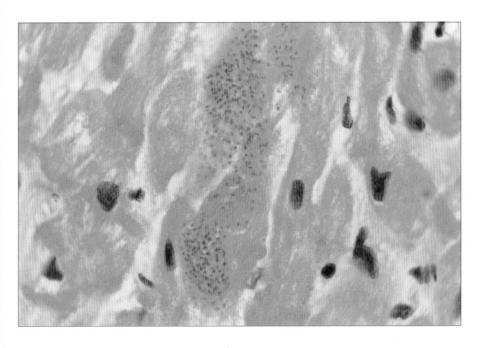

Figure 12.2
High-power view of toxoplasma cyst in a myocyte. No surrounding inflammatory infiltrate is present.

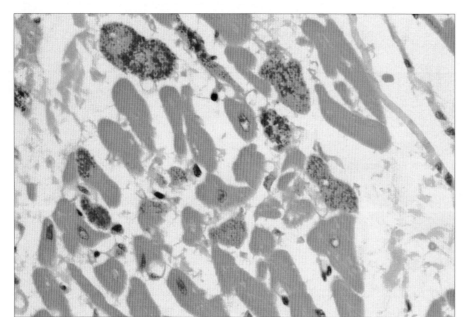

Figure 12.3
Endomyocardial biopsy high-power showing mitochondrial calcification in ischemia, not to be confused with toxoplasmosis (Fig. 12.1).

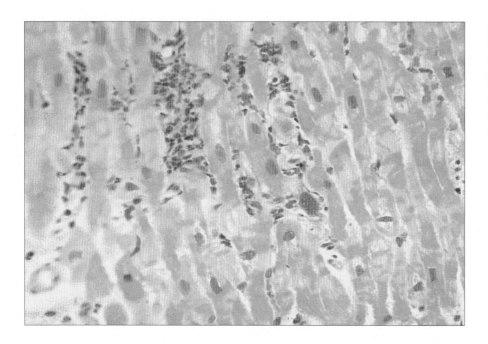

Figure 12.4
Endomyocardial biopsies, medium-power showing cytomegalovirus (CMV) myocarditis. Compared with rejection the infiltrate includes some neutrophils. No inclusions are seen in this field, but the presence of neutrophils should alert the pathologist to the possibility of CMV.

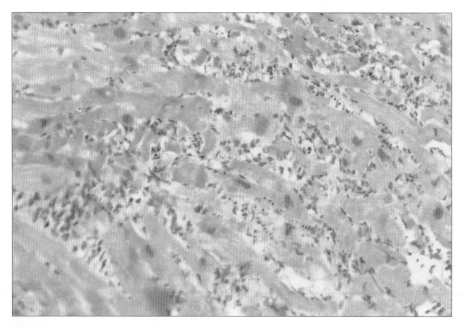

Figure 12.5
Interstitial infiltrate in which neutrophils predominate. There are nuclear inclusions in several mycytes. CMV myocarditis with obvious inclusions is very rare.

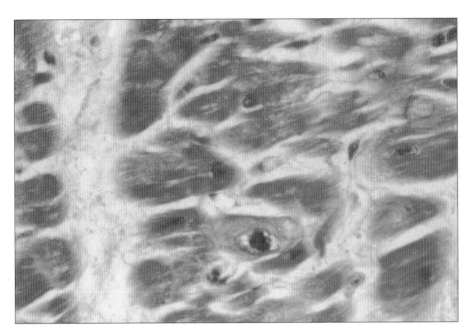

Figure 12.6
No infiltrate is seen: however a myocyte contains a nuclear inclusion. Immunohistochemistry was positive in this case. Similar nuclear changes can be seen in degenerative myocytes.

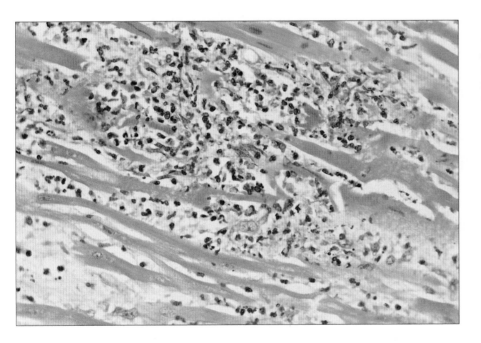

Figure 12.7
Medium-power view of an intramyocardial abscess in a case of disseminated *Aspergillus* infection in a cardiac transplant recipient. Some hyphal material can just be made out amongst the infiltrate.

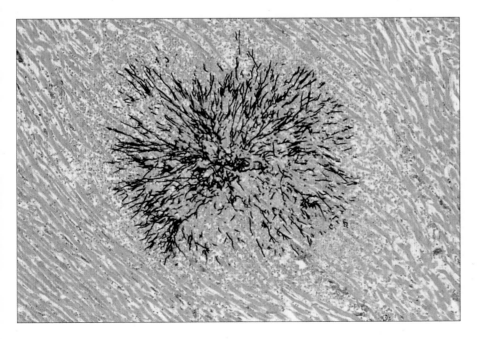

Figure 12.8
Medium-power view showing *Aspergillus* hyphae in myocardium in another case of disseminated *Aspergillus* infection in a cardiac transplant recipient. It is important to carry out a Grocott's silver stain as in this case if fungal infection is suspected.

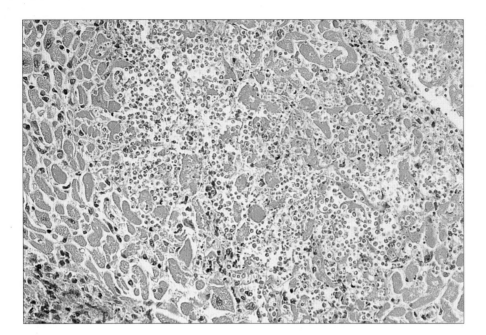

Figure 12.9
Medium-power view showing spores of *Candida* in the myocardium of a heavily immunosuppressed cardiac transplant recipient.

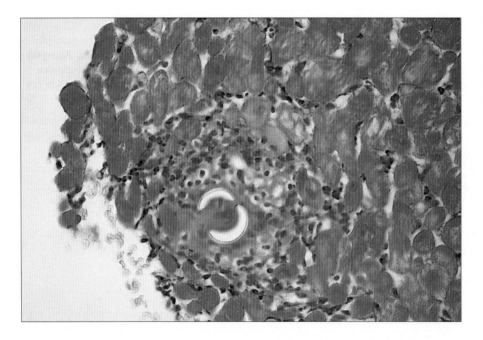

Figure 12.10
High-power view of a fortuitous biopsy from a cardiac transplant recipient who was a farmer in the Central Valley in California and who developed disseminated coccidiomycosis infection on immunosuppression.

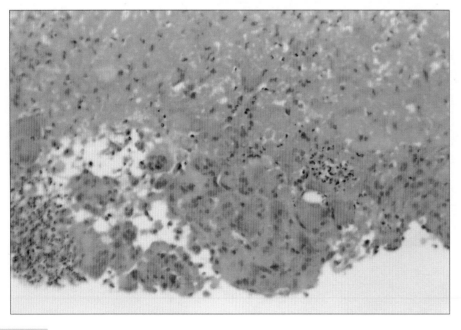

Figure 12.11
High-power showing acute and granulomatous inflammation in the endocardium in a heavily immunosuppressed cardiac transplant recipient.

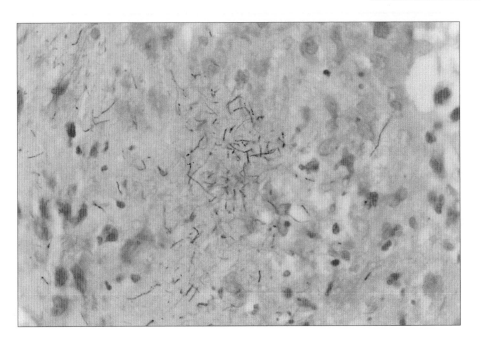

Figure 12.12
Gram stain of an adjacent section to Fig. 12.10, showing branching Gram-positive bacilli in keeping with *Nocardia* infection. This was proven on culture in life and on subsequent autopsy.

FURTHER READING

Cohnert TR, Kemnitz J, Haverich A, Dralle H. Myocardial calcification following heart transplantation. *J Heart Transplant* 1986;5:332–5.

Everett JP, Herschbergen RE, Norman DJ *et al*. Prolonged cytomegalovirus infection with uraemia is associated with development of cardiac allograft vasculopathy. *J Heart Lung Transplant* 1992; 11:S133–7.

Grattan MT, Moreno-Cabral CE, Starnes VA, Oyer PE, Stinson EB, Shumway NE. Cytomegalovirus infection is associated with cardiac allograft rejection and atherosclerosis. *JAMA* 1989;261:3561–6.

Holliman R, Johnson J, Saber D, Cary N, Wreghitt T. Diagnosis of toxoplasma infection in cardiac transplant recipients using the polymerase chain reaction. *J Clin Pathol* 1992;45:931–2.

Hutter JA, Scott P, Wreghitt T, Higenbottam T, Wallwork J. The importance of cytomegalovirus in heart–lung transplant recipients. *Chest* 1989;95:627–31.

Janner D, Bork J, Baum M, Chinnock R. *Pneumocystis carinii* pneumonia in infants after heart transplantation. *J Heart Lung Transplant* 1996;15:755–63.

Kanj SS, Welty-Wolf K, Madden J *et al*. Fungal infections in lung and heart–lung transplant recipients. Report of 9 cases and review of literature. *Medicine (Baltimore)* 1996;75:142–56.

Linder LJ. Infection as a complication of heart transplantation. *J Heart Transplant* 1988;7:390–4.

McDonald K, Rector TS, Braunlin EA, Kubo SH, Olivari MT. Association of coronary artery disease in cardiac transplant recipients with cytomegalovirus infection. *Am J Cardiol* 1989;64:359–62.

Stovin PG, Wreghitt T, English T, Wallwork J. Lack of association between cytomegalovirus infection of heart and rejection-like inflammation. *J Clin Pathol* 1989;42:81–3.

Wreghitt TG, Hackim M, Gray JJ *et al*. Toxoplasmosis in heart and heart-lung transplant recipients. The Papworth Hospital Series. *J Clin Pathol* 1989; 42:194–9.

SECTION THIRTEEN
LYMPHOPROLIFERATIVE DISEASE

Post-transplant lymphoproliferative disease (PTLPD) may occasionally be seen on endomyocardial biopsies either in patients known to have the disease elsewhere or as a first presentation/unsuspected finding. This condition is covered in detail in the lung section (Section 31) where it occurs with frequent involvement of the graft itself.

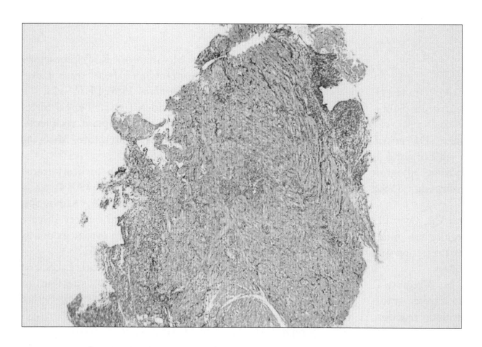

Figure 13.1
Low-power view of an endomyocardial biopsy showing extensive infiltration by lymphoproliferative disease.

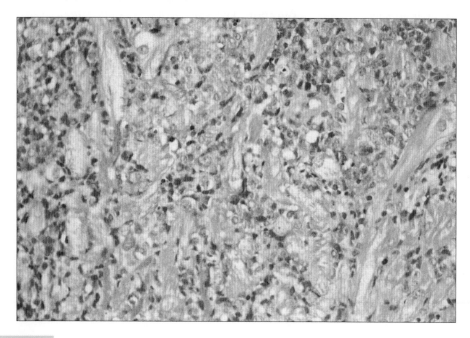

Figure 13.2
High-power view of the infiltrate shown in Fig. 13.1. The obvious neoplastic nature of the infiltrate of large highly atypical cells is seen at higher magnification.

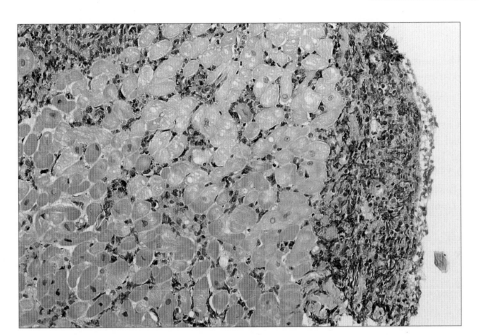

Figure 13.3
Another case of lymphoproliferative disease with conspicuous involvement of both the endocardium and deeper myocardium. Infiltrating cells are larger than seen in a rejection infiltrate.

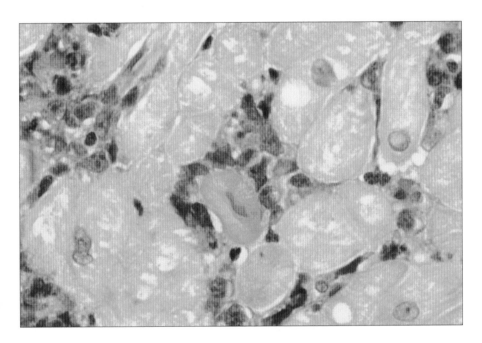

Figure 13.4
Higher power view of the myocardium of the case shown in Fig. 13.3, demonstrating the obviously atypical nature of the infiltrate compared with rejection. Other distinguishing features are the diffuseness and intensity in the face of a lack of any obvious direct evidence of myocyte damage.

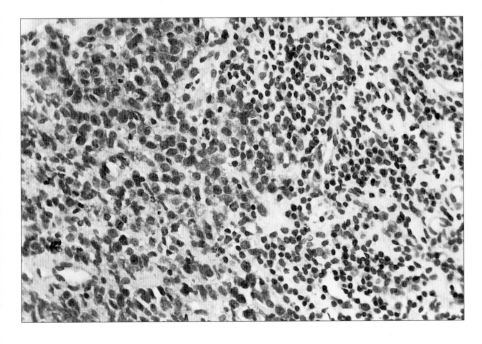

Figure 13.5
The endocardium in this case showed evidence of presumed non-neoplastic Quilty type infiltration (right-hand field) which contrasts well with the atypical neoplastic infiltrate (left-hand field).

FURTHER READING

Chadburn A, Chen JM, Hsu DJ *et al.* The morphologic and molecular genetic categories of post-transplantation lymphoproliferative disorders are clinically relevant. *Cancer* 1998;**82**:1978–87.

Chetty R, Biddolph S, Kaklamanis L, Cary N, Stewart S, Giatromanolaki A, Gatter K. bcl-2 protein is strongly expressed in post-transplant lymphoproliferative disorders. *J Pathol* 1996;**180**:254–8.

Couteil JP, McGoldrich J P, Wallwork J, English TAH. Malignant tumours after heart transplantation. *J Heart Transplant* 1990;**9**:622–6.

Fischer T, Miller M, Bott-Silverman C, Lichtin A. Post transplant lymphoproliferative disorder after cardiac transplantation. *Transplantation* 1996; **62**:1687–90.

Fischer T, Miller M, Bott-Silverman C, Lichtin A. Post transplant lymphoproliferative disease after cardiac transplantation. Two unusual variants with predominantly plasmacytoid features. *Transplantation* 1996;**62**:1687–90.

Garlicki M, Wierzbicki K. Przybylowski P *et al.* The incidence of malignancy in heart transplant recipients. *Ann Transplant* 1998;**3**:41–7.

Goldstein DJ, Austin JH, Zuech N *et al.* Carcinoma of the lung after heart transplantation. *Transplantation* 1996;**62**:772–5.

Hunt BJ, Thomas JA, Burke M, Walker H, Yacoub M, Crawford DH. Epstein–Barr virus associated Burkitt lymphoma in a heart transplant recipient. *Transplantation* 1996;**62**:869–72.

Penn I. Solid tumours in cardiac allograft recipients. *Ann Thorac Surg* 1995;**60**:1559–60.

SECTION FOURTEEN
PREVIOUS BIOPSY SITE

As cardiac transplant recipients have a large number of biopsies, sites of previous biopsies are commonly encountered, particularly early on when biopsies are most frequent.

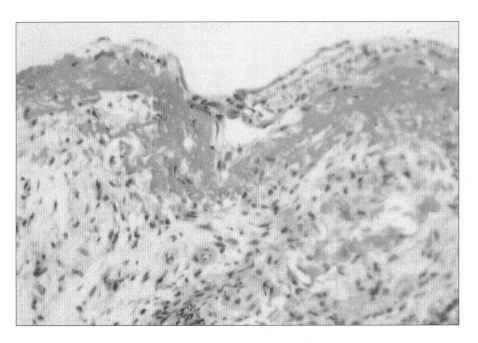

Figure 14.1
Previous biopsy site fibrinous exudate. When biopsy has occurred as here relatively recently a previous biopsy site consists of ongoing fibrinous exudate. The resulting granulation tissue must be distinguished from severe rejection which will tend to involve all fragments, though multiple fragments all showing biopsy site changes may occasionally be encountered.

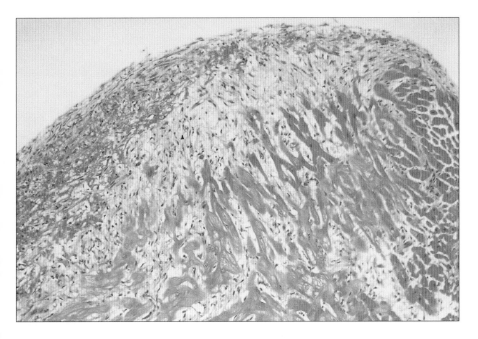

Figure 14.2
Healing of biopsy site produces edematous granulation tissue. There may be an accompanying infiltrate involving the myocardium which should not be confused with rejection.

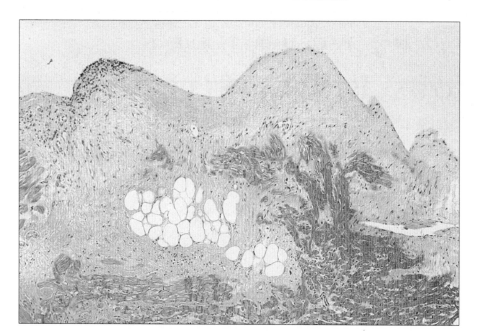

Figure 14.3
Old healed biopsy site showing replacement fibrosis and distortion of adjoining myocytes. There are a few entrapped lymphocytes within the area of scarring.

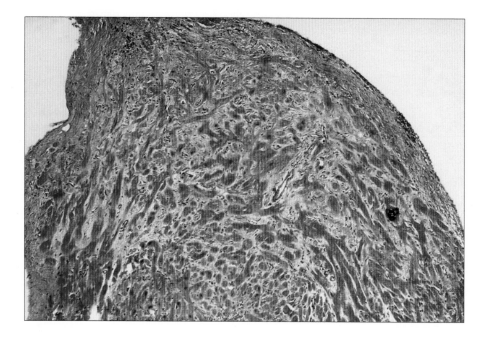

Figure 14.4
A trichrome stain helps to demonstrate the fibrosis and disarray in myocardium adjoining sites of previous biopsy.

OTHER FINDINGS –
MISCELLANEOUS

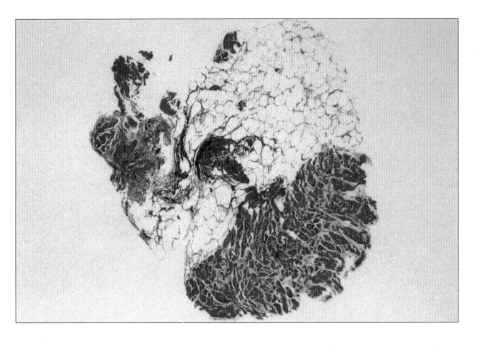

Figure 15.1
Conspicuous epicardial or intramyocardial fat may be encountered in right ventricular biopsies and is of no consequence. The fat is highlighted in this trichrome-stained section.

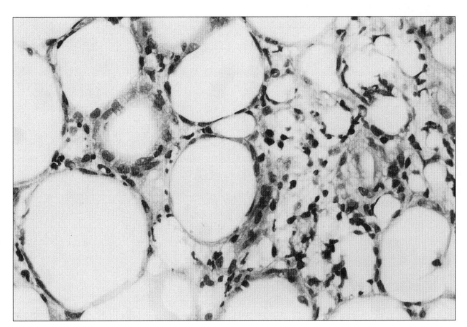

Figure 15.2
Intramyocardial fat may produce a lipogranulomatous reaction, not to be confused with rejection. Epicardial lymphocytic infiltrates may be seen and do not constitute rejection.

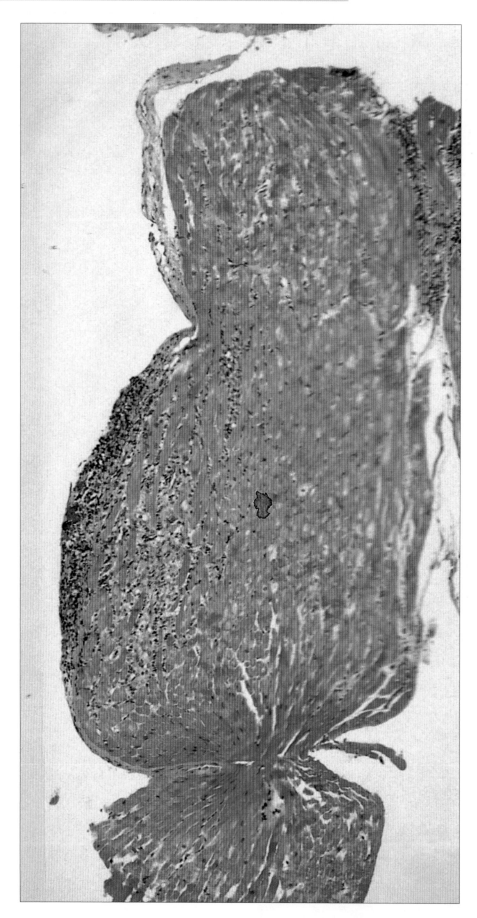

Figure 15.3
A granulomatous reaction in relation to foreign material may be seen sub-endocardially. This material may be introduced by the bioptome in a previous biopsy.

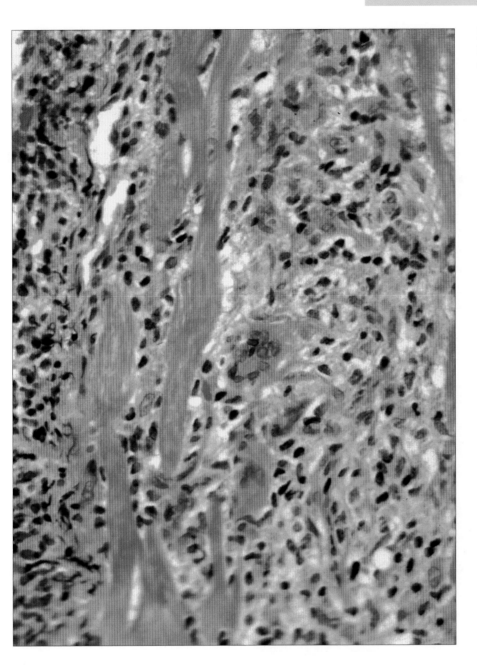

Figure 15.4
High-power view with giant cells some containing foreign material.

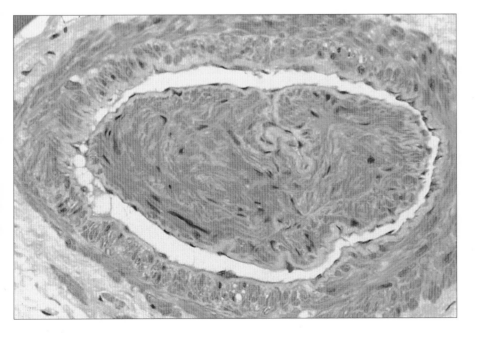

Figure 15.5
Telescoping of the media of small arteries may be seen in some biopsies and should not be confused with intimal thickening as part of graft vascular disease.

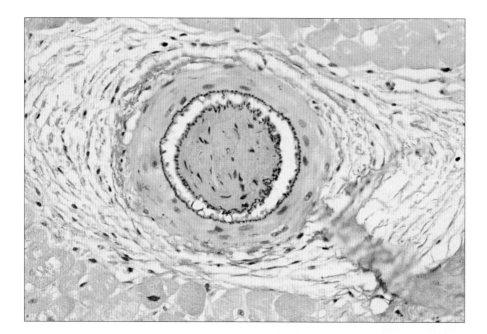

Figure 15.6
An elastic van Gieson stain demonstrates the telescoping or 'finger in glove' phenomenon.

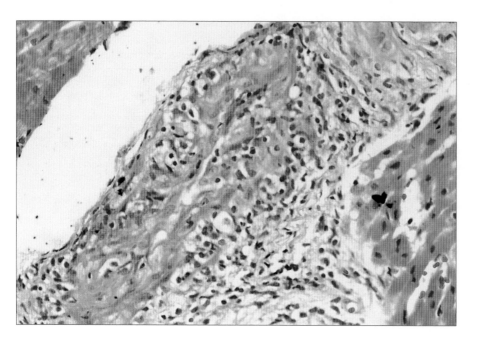

Figure 15.7
Vasculitic changes may be seen in biopsies. The changes do not fit easily into the ISHLT classification. They more commonly occur with higher grades of rejection, but when occurring alone or with only one area of damaging myocardial infiltrate can cause difficulties. Careful correlation with clinical parameters is necessary. In our institutions, we have tended to view an area of vasculitis as a focus of moderate rejection and adjusted therapy accordingly. Some studies have suggested a role in the development of chronic graft vasculopathy.

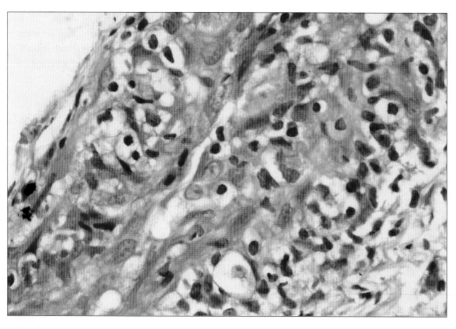

Figure 15.8
High-power view of Fig. 15.7.

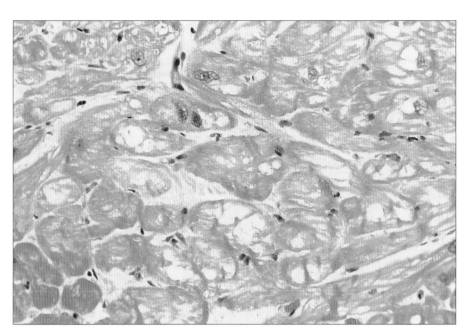

Figure 15.9
Myocyte hypertrophy occurs in transplant hearts. However, conspicuous hypertrophy with vacuolation of myocytes raises the possibility of chronic ischemia and underlying graft vasculopathy.

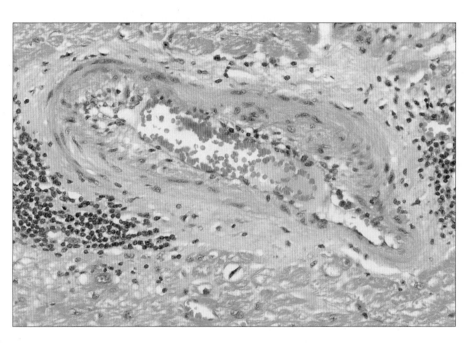

Figure 15.10
Right ventricular biopsies have a very poor diagnostic yield in relation to graft vascular disease, at least in part because the wrong size of vessels are sampled. However on occasion obvious diseased small intramyocardial arteries may be sampled such as this one. There is intimal thickening with foamy macrophages and lymphocytes.

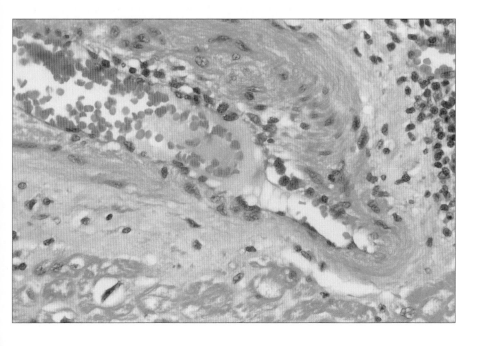

Figure 15.11
Higher power view of intimal thickening and infiltrate.

HUMORAL REJECTION

Humoral rejection is reported with different frequencies from different transplant centers and there are no agreed diagnostic criteria. Humoral rejection is associated with the *de novo* synthesis of antibodies directed against HLA antigens expressed on graft endothelium, and there may also be complement activation.

The diagnosis is usually made on the histologic criteria of endothelial swelling and vasculitis, and by the immunohistologic demonstration of the deposition of immunoglobulins and complement proteins. Some authors have suggested that staining patterns for these substances is non-specific and not diagnostically useful.

The diagnosis of humoral rejection is very rare in our institution and in most cases there is an associated cellular component which can be assessed in the normal way.

FURTHER READING

Aretz HT, Colvin RB. Endomyocardial biopsies. An early warning system for chronic transplant arteriopathy. *JAMA* 1997;**278**:1197–8.

Armstrong AT, Binkley PF, Baker PB, Myerowitz PD, Leier CV. Quantitative investigation of cardiomyocyte hypertrophy and myocardial fibrosis over 6 years after cardiac transplantation. *J Am Coll Cardiol* 1998;**32**:704–10.

Bonnaud EV, Lewis NP, Masek MA, Billingham ME. Reliability and usefulness of immunofluorescence in heart transplantation. *J Heart Lung Transplant* 1995;**14**:163–71.

Boyle JJ, Jenkins J, McKay IC, McPhaden AR, Lindop GB. An assessment of the distribution of arteries due to sectioning in endomyocardial biopsies. *J Pathol* 1997;**181**:243–6.

Conraads V, Lahaye I, Rademakers F *et al.* Cardiac graft vasculopathy: aetiologic factors and therapeutic approaches. *Acta Cardiol* 1998;**53**:37–43.

Dong C, Redenbach D, Wood S, Battistini B, Wilson JE, McManus BM. The pathogenesis of cardiac allograft vasculopathy. *Curr Opin Cardiol* 1996;**11**:183–90.

Hammond EH, Handsen JK, Spencer LS, Jensen A, Yowell RL. Immunofluorescence of endomyocardial biopsy specimens: methods and interpretation. *J Heart Lung Transplant* 1993;**12**:113–24.

Hammond EH, Yowell RJ, Price GD *et al.* Vascular rejection and its relationship to allograft coronary artery disease. *J Heart Lung Transplant* 1992;**11**:111–9.

Hammond EH, Yowell RL, Nunoda S *et al.* Vascular (humoral) rejection in heart transplantation: Pathologic Observations and Clinical Implications. *J Heart Transplant* 1989;**8**:430–43.

Higuchi M, Benvenuti L, Demarchi L, Libby P. Histologic evidence of concomitant intramyocardial and epicardial vasculitis in necropsied heart allograft. *Transplantation* 1999;**67**:1569–76

Hruban RH, Beschorner WE, Baumgartner WA *et al.* Accelerated arteriosclerosis in heart transplant recipients is associated with a T-lymphocyte-mediated endothelialitis. *Am J Pathol* 1990;**137**:871–82.

Jenkins J, Boyle JJ, Moss VA, McPhaden AR, Lindop GB. Three dimensional reconstruction of abnormal intramural coronary arteries in human cardiac allograft biopsies. *J Pathol* 1997;**181**:247–50.

Lones MA, Czer LSC, Trento A, Harasty D, Miller JM, Fishbein MC. Clinical pathology features of humoral rejection in cardiac allograft: a study of 81 consecutive patients. *J Heart Lung Transplant* 1995;**14**:151–62.

Luthringer DJ, Yamashita JT, Czer LS, Trento A, Fishbein MC. Nature and significance of epicardial lymphoid infiltrates in cardiac allografts. *J Heart Lung Transplant* 1995;**14**:537–43.

Pardo-Mindan FJ, Panizo A, Lozano MD, Herreros J, Mejia S. Role of endomyocardial biopsy in the diagnosis of chronic rejection in human heart transplantation. *Clin Transplant* 1997;**11**:426–31.

Smith SH, Kirklin JK, Geer JC, Caulfield JB, McGiffin D. Arteritis in cardiac rejection after transplantation. *Am J Cardiol* 1987;**59**:1171–3.

Winters GL, Schoen FJ. Graft arteriosclerosis-induced myocardial pathology in heart transplant recipients: predictive value of endomyocardial biopsy. *J Heart Lung Transplant* 1997;**16**:985–93.

PART 2

TRANSBRONCHIAL LUNG BIOPSIES FOR LUNG TRANSPLANT RECIPIENTS BASED ON ISHLT GRADING SYSTEM

INTRODUCTION

INTRODUCTION

When combined heart–lung transplantation was introduced as a clinical procedure, acute rejection was monitored by endomyocardial biopsy which was a well-established diagnostic procedure. However it soon became clear that the lungs in combined grafts rejected more frequently and more vigorously than the grafted hearts and there was a need to examine biopsies of lung parenchyma directly. In addition, the transplanted lung is more prone to normal and opportunistic infection, thereby widening the differential diagnosis. Transbronchial lung biopsies soon became established as the gold standard for diagnosing and grading acute pulmonary rejection and for distinguishing it from important differential diagnoses. The International Society for Heart and Lung Transplantation sponsored a workshop in 1990 for the classification and grading of lung rejection (Table 3). This working formulation aimed to be simple, easily taught and readily reproducible and also aimed to incorporate the best aspects of other grading systems in use at the time. It mainly lived up to these expectations, the major drawback being the common problem of biopsies showing concomitant pathologies, e.g. acute rejection and infection. In 1995 an expanded lung rejection study group revised the 1990 working formulation on the basis of greater experience and published data (Table 4). The revised classification is further simplified with an option

for grading of airway inflammation. Again exclusion of infection is emphasized as being essential for accurate and reproducible interpretation of lung allograft biopsies. It is also recommended that although the grading system is based on histopathologic appearances, interpretation of biopsy data should be in a clinical context for optimum patient management.

Transbronchial biopsies remain the 'gold standard' for the diagnosis of acute rejection with clinical, radiologic and immunologic techniques proving non-specific. The application of molecular methods to biopsy material studying cellular profiles, cytokines and gene expression in rejection and infection has produced few clinical benefits as yet. The correct interpretation of these novel techniques requires the morphological substrate which is only available through high quality reading of biopsy material.

There are numerous reports on the use of transbronchial biopsies in diagnosis and management of post operative complications. Biopsies can fall into three categories: clinically indicated, surveillance or follow-up biopsies. The use of surveillance biopsies has decreased in many centers without adverse effect on survival and our current practice is to use clinically directed biopsies with a single 'base-line' surveillance biopsy at approximately 28 days prior to discharge from hospital. When interpreting the high incidence of abnormalities found

---

Table 3

Working formulation for classification and grading of pulmonary rejection (1990)

Grade A: Acute rejection	
	Additional suffices
A1 Minimal	a. With evidence of bronchiolar inflammation
A2 Mild	b. Without evidence of bronchiolar inflammation
A3 Moderate	c. With large airway inflammation
A4 Severe	d. No bronchioles are present

Grade B: Active airway damage without scarring

B   1. Lymphocytic bronchitis   2. Lymphocytic bronchiolitis

No perivascular infiltrates, i.e. no A Grade

Grade C: Chronic airway damage with scarring

C   1. Bronchiolitis obliterans - subtotal   2. Bronchiolitis obliterans – total

      a. Active   a. Active

      b. Inactive   b. Inactive

i.e. differs from B by having *fibrosis*

Grade D: Chronic vascular rejection

Fibrointimal thickening of arteries and veins

Grade E: Vasculitis

Necrosis of vessel wall disproportionate to other inflammation.

From: Yousem S A *et al.* (1990).

Table 4
Working formulation for classification and grading of lung allograft rejection

A	Acute rejection
	0 Grade 0 – None
	1 Grade 1 – Minimal
	2 Grade 2 – Mild
	3 Grade 3 – Moderate
	4 Grade 4 – Severe
B*	Airway inflammation – lymphocytic bronchitis/bronchiolitis
C	Chronic airway rejection – bronchiolitis obliterans
	a. Active
	b. Inactive
D	Chronic vascular rejection – accelerated graft vascular sclerosis

*Pathologist may choose to grade B lesions
From: Yousem S A *et al.* (1996).

Box 13   Differences between acute and chronic lung rejection

Acute lung rejection
- perivascular and subendothelial mononuclear cell infiltrates
- lymphocytic bronchitis and bronchiolitis

Chronic lung rejection
- graft vascular fibroproliferative disease
- obliterative bronchiolitis

i.e. key differences are fibrosis, nature of infiltrate

Box 14   Acute lung rejection (Grade A)

Defined as perivascular infiltrates
- Intensity
- Extension
- Cellular composition
- Endothelialitis

n.b. Excludes infiltrates around vessels in airways

Box 15   Acute lung rejection (Grade A)

- Grade 0 – None
- Grade 1 – Minimal   with/without   Grade B
- Grade 2 – Mild   airway inflammation
- Grade 3 – Moderate
- Grade 4 – Severe

Box 16   Recommendations

1. Five pieces alveolated parenchyma with bronchioles
2. More samples required to diagnose OB
3. Minimum three levels H & E
4. Connective tissue and silver stains
5. Review of previous biopsies

---

in surveillance biopsies including significant grades of acute rejection and active infection, it should be realized that some of the patients were not truly asymptomatic at the time of biopsy. However the use of these routine biopsies and follow-up biopsies has contributed to the knowledge and understanding of the transplanted lung.

The treatment threshold for acute lung rejection is usually A2 and higher, but this is not a hard and fast rule.

Grade A1, A2 and A3 can all be clinically silent and there is evidence that Grade 1 and some Grade A2 acute rejection can resolve without augmented immunosuppression. Some Grade A2 acute rejection will progress, but there are no definite predictive features. As the lung suffers a high incidence of acute rejection amongst solid organ grafts, studies with appropriate controls are difficult to perform and the incidence and significance of clinically silent acute rejection remains uncertain.

ADEQUACY OF SPECIMENS

Transbronchial biopsy is the current gold standard allograft evaluation and it is essential that adequate specimens are obtained for diagnosis. The lung rejection study group requires at least five pieces of alveolated lung parenchyma with bronchioles and ideally containing greater than 100 alveoli. In practical terms this means the bronchoscopist should submit more than five pieces in order to provide this minimum number of parenchymal biopsies as some fragments may consist only of bronchial wall or even pleural tissue. Also, if obliterative bronchiolitis is considered likely, the number of pieces should be further increased to enhance the yield of small airways. The biopsy fragments are gently agitated in formalin to inflate them and processed according to urgency, a 2-hour schedule being more than adequate for the most urgent specimens. Careful handling is essential to avoid crush and other artefacts (*see* Appendix I).

Sections from at least three levels of the paraffin block should be examined with H & E stains which is a *minimum* standard. Many centers including our own examine multiple serial sections of the pulmonary biopsies, thus increasing the total area of parenchyma examined. Connective tissue stains are mandatory for the identification of airway, vascular and parenchymal fibrosis. Silver stains are mandatory for diagnosis of fungi and *Pneumocystis* as the latter can be an exact mimic of acute rejection. This range of stains can be supplemented with histochemical, immunohistochemical or molecular techniques for further diagnosis or research purposes.

Box 17 Differential diagnosis of perivascular and interstitial infiltrates

Perivascular and interstitial mononuclear infiltrates are not specific for acute rejection, and other conditions may simulate or mimic alloreactive injury
- Cytomegalovirus pneumonitis
- *Pneumocystic carinii* pneumonia
- Post-transplantation lymphoproliferative disease
- Bronchial associated lymphoid tissue
- Previous biopsy sites
- Recurrent primary disease, for example, sarcoidosis
- Ischemia (preservation injury)
- Drug reaction

FURTHER READING

Bando K, Paradis IL, Komatsu K *et al*. Analysis of time-dependent risks for infection, rejection and death after pulmonary transplantation. *J Thorac Cardiovasc Surg* 1995;**109**:49–59.

Bergin CJ, Castellino RA, Blank N, Berry GJ, Sibley RK, Starnes VA. Acute lung rejection after heart–lung transplantation: Correlation of findings on chest radiographs with lung biopsy results. *AJR* 1990;**155**:23–27.

Boehler A, Vogt P, Zollinger A, Weder W, Speich R. Prospective study of the value of transbronchial lung biopsy after lung transplantation. *Eur Respir J* 1996;**9**:658–62.

Briffa N, Morris RE. New immunosuppressive regimens in lung transplantation. *Eur Respir J* 1997;**10**:2630–37.

Cazzadori A, Di Perri G, Todeschini G *et al*. Transbronchial biopsy in the diagnosis of pulmonary infiltrates in immunocompromised patients. *Chest* 1995;**107**:101–6.

Chan CC, Abi-Saleh WJ, Arroliga AC *et al*. Diagnostic yield and therapeutic impact of flexible bronchoscopy in lung transplant recipients. *J Heart Lung Transplant* 1996;**15**:196–205.

Clelland CA, Higenbottam TW, Stewart S, Scott JP, Wallwork J. The histological changes in transbronchial biopsy after treatment of acute lung rejection in heart–lung recipients. *J Pathol* 1990;**161**:105–112.

Day JD, Hutchins GM, Hruban RH. Grading pulmonary rejection: a proposal for a simplified system. *J Heart Lung Transplant* 1994;**13**:734–7.

de Blic J, Peuchmaur M, Carnot F *et al*. Rejection in lung transplantation – an immunohistochemical study of transbronchial biopsies. *Transplantation* 1992;**54**:639–44.

De Hoyos A, Chamberlain D, Schwartzman R *et al*. Prospective assessment of a standardised pathologic grading system for acute rejection in lung transplantation. *Chest* 1993;**103**:1813–18.

Gilman MJ, Wang KP. Transbronchial lung biopsy in sarcoidosis – an approach to determine the optimal number of biopsies. *Am Rev Respir Dis* 1980; **122**:721–4.

Guilinger RA, Paradis IL, Dauber JH *et al*. The importance of bronchoscopy with transbronchial biopsy and bronchoalveolar lavage in the management of lung transplant recipients. *Am J Respir Crit Care Med* 1995;**152**:2037–43.

Harjula AJL, Baldwin JC, Glanville AR *et al*. Human leukocyte antigen compatibility in heart–lung transplantation. *J Heart Transplant* 1987;**6**:162–6.

Higenbottam TW, Stewart S, Penketh AR, Wallwork J. Transbronchial lung biopsy for the diagnosis of rejection in heart–lung transplant patients. *Transplantation* 1988;**46**:532–39.

Higenbottam TW, Stewart S, Wallwork J. Transbronchial lung biopsy to diagnose lung rejection and infection of heart–lung transplants. *Transplant Proc* 1988;**20**:767–9.

Higenbottam TW, Stewart S. Transbronchial lung biopsy in the diagnosis of rejection of the transplanted lung. In: *Heart and Heart-lung transplantation*. (Ed J Wallwork). 1989; pp. 523–32. W B Saunders, Philadelphia.

Hruban RH, Beschorner WE, Baumgartner WA *et al*. Evidence that the expression of class II MHC antigens is not diagnostic of lung allograft rejection. *Transplantation* 1989;**48**:529–30.

Hunt JB, Stewart S, Cary N, Wreghitt TG, Higenbottam TW, Wallwork J. Evaluation of the International Society for Heart Transplantation grading of pulmonary rejection in 100 consecutive biopsies. *Transplant Int* 1992;**5**:S249–S251.

Hutter JA, Stewart S, Higenbottam TW, Scott JP, Wallwork J. The characteristic histological changes associated with rejection in heart-lung transplant recipients. *Transplant Proc* 1989;**21**:435–6.

Keenan RJ, Bruzzone P, Paradis IL *et al*. Similarity of pulmonary rejection patterns among heart-lung and double lung transplant recipients. *Transplantation* 1991;**51**:176–80.

Kesten S, Chamberlain D, Maurer J. Yield of surveillance transbronchial biopsies performed beyond two years after lung transplantation. *J Heart Lung Transplant* 1996;**15**:384–8.

Kukafka DS, O'Brien GM, Furukawa S, Criner GJ. Surveillance bronchoscopy in lung transplant recipients. *Chest* 1997;**111**:377–81.

Loubeyre P, Revel D, Delignette A, Loire R, Morex J-F. High-resolution computed tomographic findings associated with histologically diagnosed acute lung rejection in heart–lung transplant recipients. *Chest* 1995;**107**:132–38.

Medina LS, Siegel MJ, Bejaranmo PA, Glazer HS, Anderson DJ, Mallory Jr GB. Pediatric lung transplantation: radiographic histopathologic correlation. *Radiology* 1993;**187**:807–10.

Medina LS, Siegel MJ, Glazer HS *et al*. Diagnosis of pulmonary complications associated with lung transplantation in children: value of CT vs histological studies. *AJR* 1994;**164**:969–74.

Millet B, Higenbottam TW, Flower CDR, Stewart S, Wallwork J. The radiographic appearances of infection and acute rejection of the lung after heart–lung transplantation. *Am Rev Respir Dis* 1989;**140**:62–7.

O'Donovan PB. Imaging of complications of lung transplantation. *RadioGraphics* 1993;**13**:787–96.

Pomerance A, Madden B, Burke MM, Yacoub MH. Transbronchial biopsy in heart and lung transplantation: Clinicopathologic correlations. *J Heart Lung Transplant* 1995;**14**:761–73.

Scott WC, Haverich A, Billingham ME, Dawkins KD, Jamieson SW. Lethal rejection of the lung without significant cardiac rejection in primate heart–lung allotransplants. *J Heart Transplant* 1984;**4**:33–9.

Shreeniwas R, Schulman LL, Narasimhan M, McGregor CC, Marboe CC. Adhesion molecules (E-Selectin and ICAM-1) in pulmonary allograft rejection. *Chest* 1996;**110**:1143–9.

Sibley RK, Berry GJ, Tazelaar HD *et al.* The role of transbronchial biopsies in the management of lung transplant recipients. *J Heart Lung Transplant* 1993;**12**:308–24.

Snover DC. Clinically silent rejection: what's in a name, anyway? *Hum Pathol* 1996;**27**:319–20.

Starnes VA, Theodore J, Oyer PE *et al.* Evaluation of heart-lung transplant recipients with prospective, serial transbronchial biopsies and pulmonary function studies. *J Thor Cardiovasc Surg* 1989; **98**:683–90.

Starnes VA, Theodore J, Oyer PE *et al.* Pulmonary infiltrates after heart–lung transplantation: evaluation by serial transbronchial biopsies. *J Thor Cardiovasc Surg* 1989;**98**:945–50.

Stewart S. Pathology of lung transplantation. In: *Practical pulmonary pathology.* (Ed MN Sheppard). 1995; pp. 88–109. Edward Arnold, London.

Stewart S. Lung transplantation. In: *Morphology of transplantation*, Chapter 11. (Eds S Thiru, H Waldman). 2000; pp. 320–52. Blackwell Scientific Publications, Oxford.

Stewart S. The pathology of lung transplantation. *Sem Diag Pathol* 1992;**9**:210–19.

Sundaresan S, Cooper JD. Lung transplantation. *Ann Thorac Surg* 1998;**65**:293–4.

Tazelaar HD. Perivascular inflammation in pulmonary infections: Implications for the diagnosis of lung rejection. *J Heart Lung Transplant* 1991;**10**:437–41.

Trulock EP, Ettinger NA, Brunt EM, Pasque MK, Kaiser LR, Cooper JD. The role of transbronchial lung biopsy in the treatment of lung transplant recipients. *Chest* 1992;**102**:1049–54.

Trulock EP. Lung transplantation. *Am J Respir Crit Care Med* 1997;**155**:789–818.

Yousem SA, Berry GJ, Brunt EM et al. A working formulation for the standardization of nomenclature in the diagnosis of heart and lung rejection: Lung rejection study group. *J Heart Transplant* 1990;**9**:593–601.

Yousem SA, Berry GJ, Cagle PT et al. A Revision of the 1990 Working Formulation for the Classification of Lung Allograft Rejection. *J Heart Lung Transplant* 1996;**15**:1–15.

Yousem SA, Curley JM, Dauber JA et al. HLA class II antigen expression in human heart-lung allografts. *Transplantation* 1990;**49**:991–5.

Yousem SA, Martin T, Paradis IL, Keenan R, Griffiths BP. Can immunohistological analysis of transbronchial biopsy specimens predict responder status in early acute rejection of lung allografts? *Hum Pathol* 1994;**25**:525–9.

Yousem SA. Significance of clinically silent untreated mild acute cellular rejection in lung allograft recipients. *Hum Pathol* 1996;**27**:269–73.

Yousem SA. The potential role of mast cells in lung allograft rejection. *Hum Pathol* 1997;**28**:179–82.

SECTION SIXTEEN
GRADE 0 REJECTION
(NO ACUTE REJECTION)

This grade denotes biopsies showing either no evidence of cellular infiltration or extremely sparse mononuclear cell infiltrates. These are not particularly perivascular and are not considered pathologically significant.

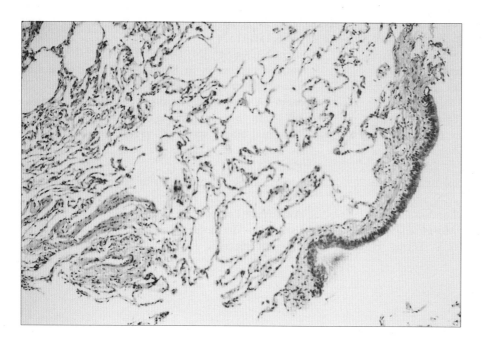

Figure 16.1
Normal transbronchial biopsy of a transplanted lung showing no significant abnormality of mucosa or parenchyma.

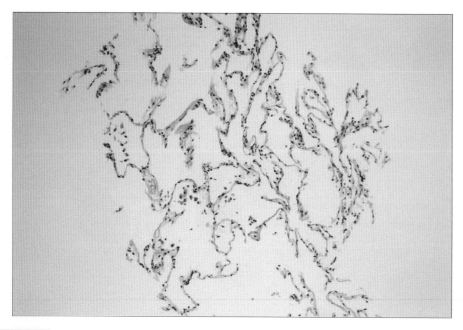

Figure 16.2
Normal parenchyma of a transplanted lung shows no evidence of inflammation. Alveolar spaces are devoid of cells and exudate.

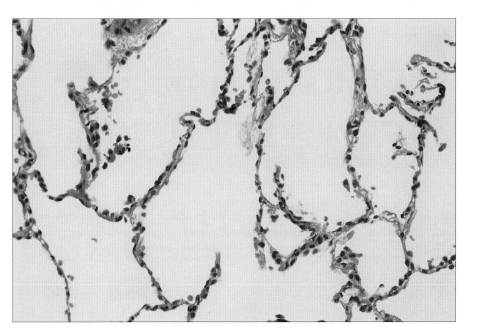

Figure 16.3
Higher power view of entirely normal parenchyma.

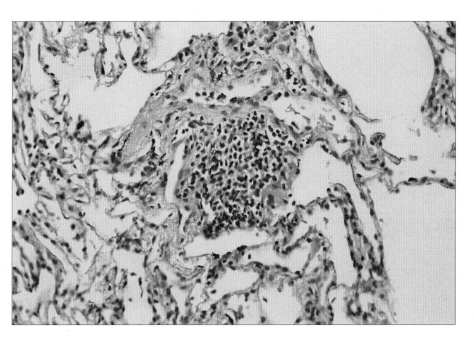

Figure 16.4
High-power view of the only abnormality present in an adequate biopsy series. This non-specific mononuclear cell infiltrate is not surrounding vessel and is composed of a small mature lymphocyte. Biopsies with this appearance should be regarded as negative for acute rejection, i.e. A0.

SECTION SEVENTEEN
GRADE A1 REJECTION
(MINIMAL ACUTE REJECTION)

This grade shows scattered infrequent perivascular mononuclear cell infiltrates which are not obvious at scanning magnification. The blood vessels, particularly venules, are cuffed by mature lymphocytes usually 2–3 cells in thickness with occasional plasmacytoid and transformed lymphocytes admixed.

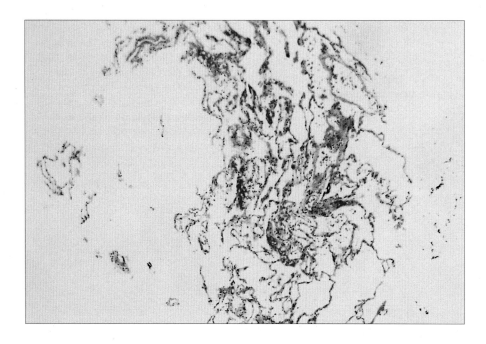

Figure 17.1
Scanning magnification of transbronchial biopsy shows no evidence of perivascular infiltrates.

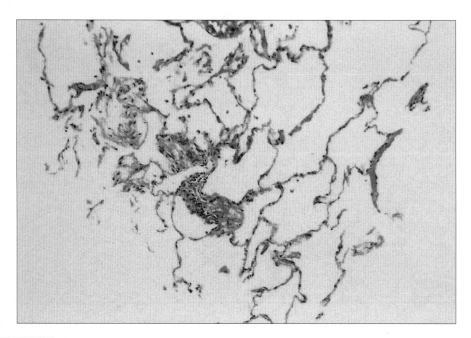

Figure 17.2
Higher power view reveals a minimum perivascular mononuclear cell infiltrate of Grade A1 rejection.

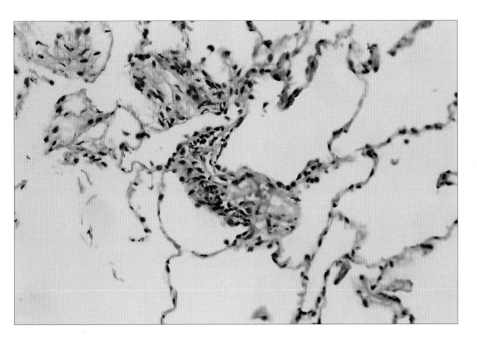

Figure 17.3
Highest power shows perivascular infiltrate with features characteristics of A1 rejection. A single eosinophil is seen.

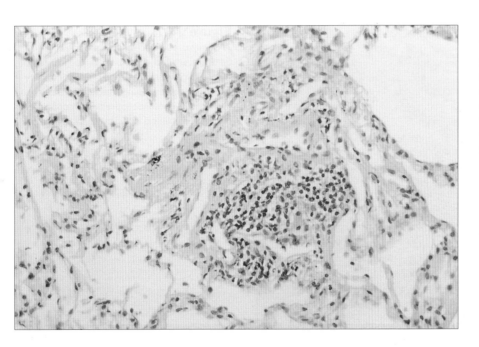

Figure 17.4
This perivascular infiltrate was not visible on scanning magnification. It consists of mature small lymphocytes only, with no evidence of endothelialitis and occurs in a background of entirely normal lung parenchyma. This was the only infiltrate in the entire biopsy series, but unlike Fig. 16.4 is clearly perivascular in distribution.

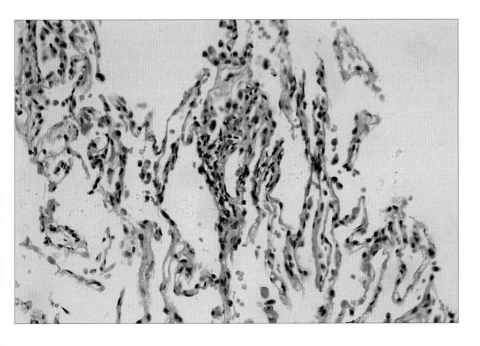

Figure 17.5
A transbronchial biopsy showing a minor mononuclear cell infiltrate around a thin-walled vessel in the center of the field. The endothelium is unremarkable. A few hemosiderin-containing macrophages are present in adjacent air spaces only.

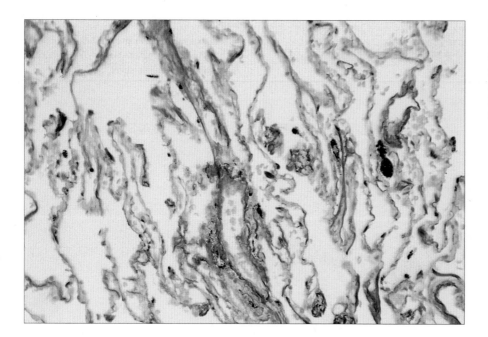

Figure 17.6
Combined Perls' – elastic van Gieson's staining shows hemosiderin deposition at the site of the infiltrate in Fig. 17.5. This A1 minimal rejection was present in a follow-up biopsy to previous treated A2 mild rejection.

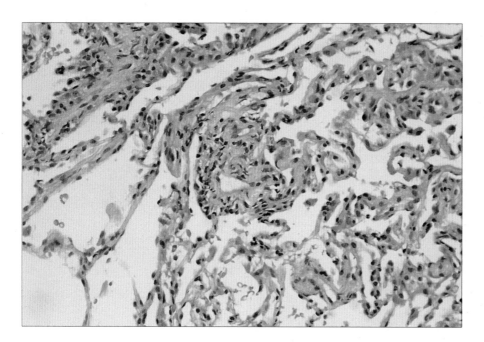

Figure 17.7
A minimal perivascular mononuclear cell infiltrate around the vessel in the center of the field consistent with A1 rejection. The patient recovered lung function without augmented immunosuppression, confirming the lack of clinical significance of this subtle abnormality.

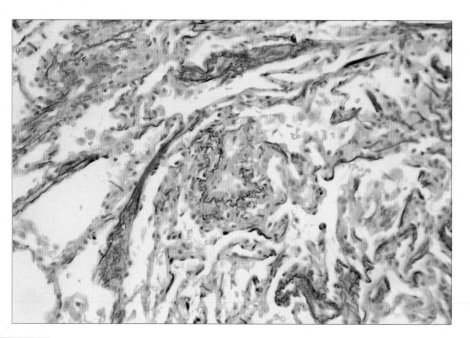

Figure 17.8
Elastic van Gieson's staining confirms the distribution of the scanty mononuclear infiltrate around the vessel of Fig. 17.7 with some hyperplastic endothelial cells. Lesions of this type are not visible at scanning magnification.

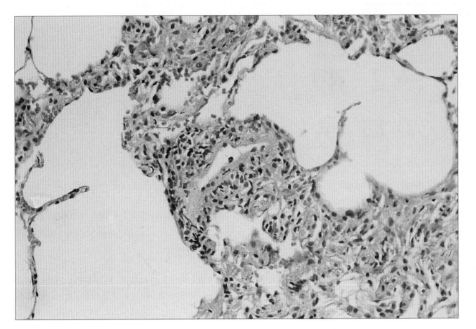

Figure 17.9
This single perivascular focus of infiltration by mononuclear cells was present in an adequate biopsy series. Although just visible at scanning magnification it is more in keeping with A1 than A2 rejection in terms of cellular composition, intensity and frequency of infiltrate. This biopsy represents the boundary between A1 and A2 acute rejection with possible intimitis. A further serial did not reveal any more infiltrates and the asymptomatic patient remained well without need for augmented immunosuppression. Biopsies like this at the treatment threshold should be assessed in terms of adequacy of parenchyma and deeper serials may be necessary to reassure or provide evidence for a higher grade.

Box 18 Grade A1 (minimal) acute rejection

- Not visible at scanning magnification
- Infrequent scattered perivascular infiltrates
- Venules particularly
- 2–3 cells thick in vessel adventitia
- Small lymphocytes, plasmacytoid

GRADE A2 REJECTION
(MILD ACUTE REJECTION)

In this grade more frequent perivascular mononuclear infiltrates surrounding venules and arterioles are easily identified at low magnification. Compared with Grade A1, there is a larger proportion of activated lymphocytes and plasmacytoid lymphocytes together with macrophages and eosinophils. Small round mature lymphocytes may however still predominate. Grade A2 rejection shows subendothelial infiltration with hyperplasia of the overlying endothelium. This lesion is known as 'endothelialitis' or 'intimitis'. The perivascular interstitium may be expanded by the inflammatory cell infiltrate, but there is no extension into adjacent alveolar septa or air spaces.

A solitary perivascular mononuclear infiltrate seen in a biopsy series demonstrating these histologic features would also be included in Grade A2 rejection. With adequate transbronchial samples and biopsies being obtained prior to any enhanced immunosuppression, this is an uncommon finding.

Box 19   Grade A2 (mild) acute rejection

- Easily seen at low magnification
- Activated lymphocytes, small lymphocytes, some plasmacytoid, macrophages, eosinophils
- Endothelialitis present
- May *expand* vascular adventitia
- Lymphocytic bronchiolitis may co-exist

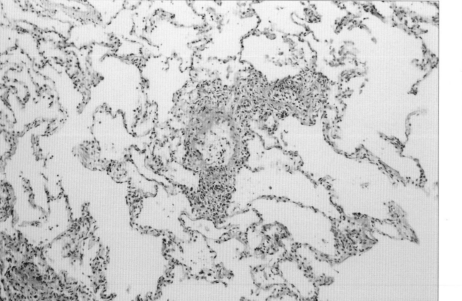

Figure 18.1
This dense perivascular infiltrate was easily visible at scanning magnification. The perivascular adventitia is expanded by mononuclear cells. There is a sharp cut-off between this adventitia and the adjacent alveolar septa and spaces which are clear of inflammation.

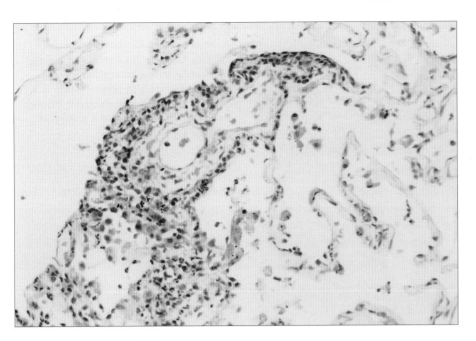

Figure 18.2
This perivascular infiltrate consists of circumferential cuffing by mononuclear cells including small and large lymphocytes with very occasional polymorphs. Eosinophils are not present. The endothelium shows hyperplasia of lining cells with scanty adherent lymphocytes indicating early endothelialitis. The adjacent airspaces are free from significant infiltrate and there is no extension of the inflammatory cells beyond the perivascular adventitia which is slightly expanded.

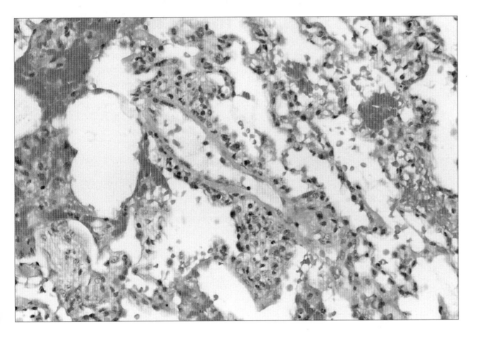

Figure 18.3
A perivascular infiltrate consisting mainly of large lymphocytes with occasional eosinophils and evidence of endothelialitis. There is some hyperplasia of alveolar epithelial cells together with hemorrhage and intra-alveolar macrophages. These additional features do not appear to be related to the acute rejection as the infiltrate is confined to the perivascular adventitia. Further serial section of the transbronchial biopsies in cases like this are helpful to exclude foci of acute rejection greater than Grade 2 elsewhere. A prompt response was made to augmented immunosuppression.

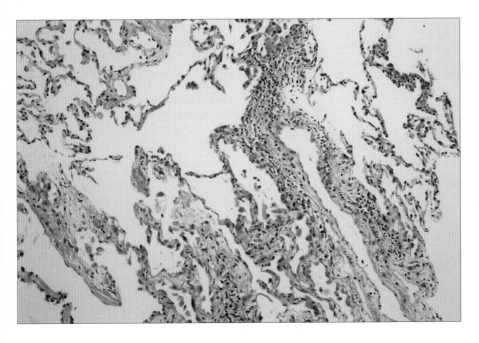

Figure 18.4
Low-power transbronchial biopsy showing perivascular infiltrate which in the plane of section involves approximately two-thirds of the vessel circumference. The presence of an intense endothelialitis is clearly seen at low-power.

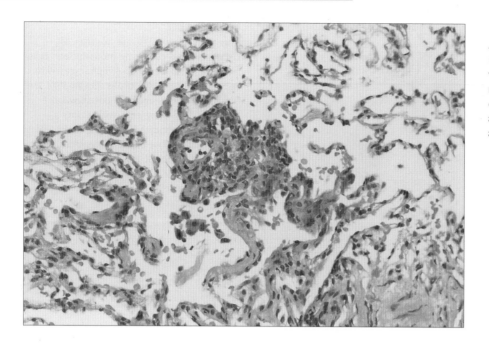

Figure 18.5
A dense perivascular mononuclear cell infiltrate following the contour of a vessel with cuffing. A few hemosiderin-laden macrophages are also present which is a common finding in lung transplant biopsies and should not influence the grading of acute rejection.

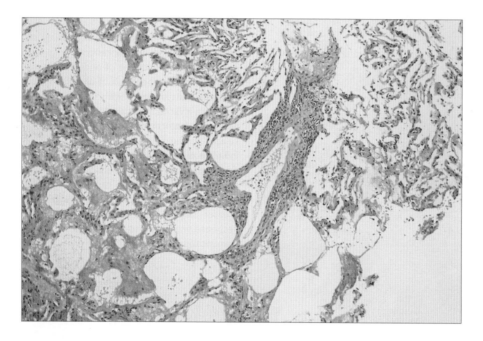

Figure 18.6
Transbronchial biopsy with a single perivascular infiltrate not involving alveolar walls, but slightly expanding the perivascular adventitia which becomes more noticeable.

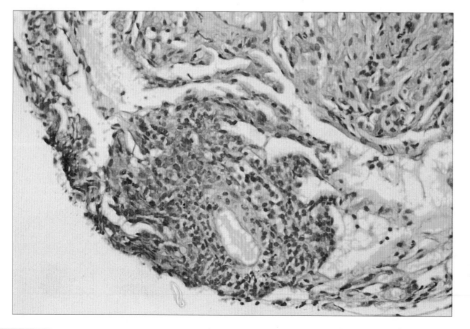

Figure 18.7
Transbronchial biopsy showing a perivascular infiltrate with expansion of the adventitial space, but no involvement of alveolar walls. There is marked endothelialitis with parallel rows of mononuclear cells within the intimal layer.

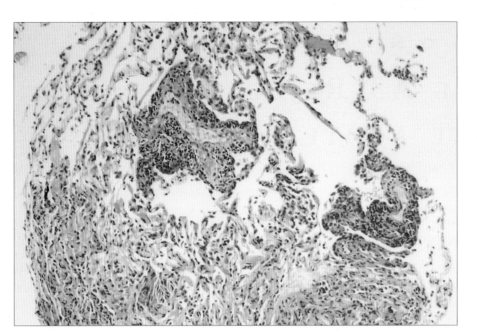

Figure 18.8
Low-power view of a patient with A2 mild rejection showing several foci of inflammatory cell infiltration centered on vessels. At low-power it is a localized process with a suggestion of involvement of perivascular alveolar walls. This is at the boundary of A2 to A3 acute rejection and is clearly at or above the usual treatment threshold of A2.

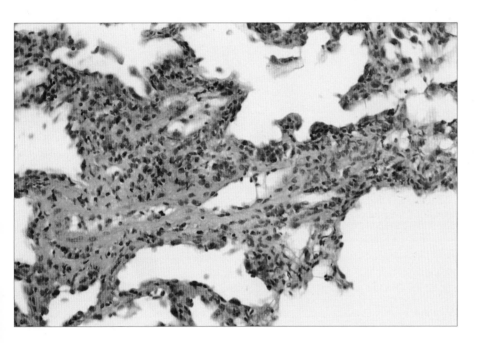

Figure 18.9
High-power view of one of these infiltrates confirms the severity of the inflammation with a high proportion of eosinophils. Endothelialitis is also present. Grade A2 rejection and above are causes of eosinophilic infiltrates. It is wise however to exclude other causes of eosinophilia, e.g. *Aspergillus* or *Pseudomonas*. These were not found in this case and a swift response to augmented immunosuppression was achieved.

GRADE A3 REJECTION (MODERATE ACUTE REJECTION)

In this grade the infiltrates are denser and more frequent than in A2 with conspicuous endothelialitis. Eosinophils and neutrophils are also more common. The defining feature of A3 acute rejection is the extension of this inflammatory infiltrate beyond the perivascular adventitia into alveolar septa and air spaces.

Infiltrating cells and increased numbers of alveolar macrophages are commonly seen in the adjacent alveoli. Similar septal infiltration of peribronchiolar infiltrates may also be seen. Grade A3 rejection is a focal process with some areas of normal parenchyma identified in the biopsy fragments.

Box 20 Grade A3 (moderate) acute rejection

- Obvious infiltrates like Grade A2 but cells extend into interstitium
- Eosinophils and neutrophils more common
- Endothelialitis usually seen
- Alveolar macrophages and alveolar epithelial cell hyperplasia

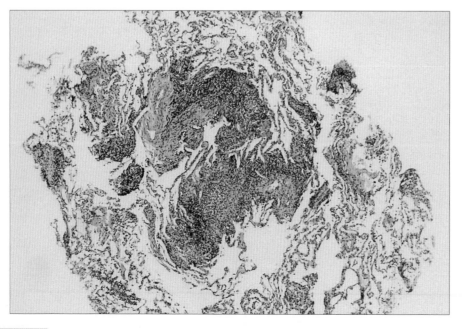

Figure 19.1
This low-power view of a transbronchial biopsy with grade A3 rejection shows dense inflammatory infiltrate centered on vessels and following their contours in the biopsy. The process is focal with remaining areas of uninvolved parenchyma. In addition to the dense infiltrates around the central vessels of the biopsy smaller infiltrates are noted at the periphery which are nonetheless readily identifiable as perivascular at this scanning power.

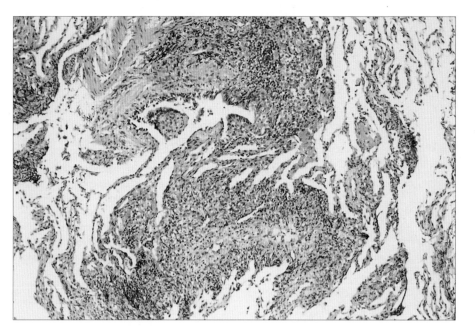

Figure 19.2
A higher power view of the same biopsy clearly shows the involvement of perivascular alveolar septa as the inflammatory infiltrate percolates out into the interstitium. The infiltrate is also contiguous with a similar infiltrate in the wall of the adjacent bronchiole which shows inflammatory cells in the subepithelial tissue. There are also areas of relatively normal parenchyma which is a useful distinction from the diffuse process of Grade A4 severe rejection.

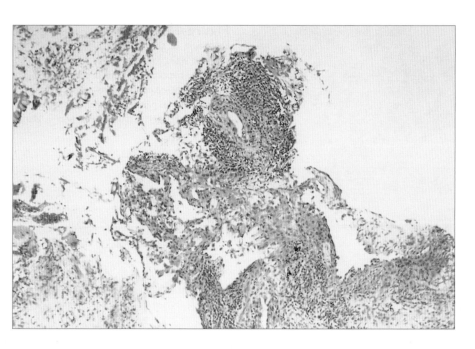

Figure 19.3
A dense perivascular infiltrate with endothelial involvement visible at low-power with extension of infiltrate into adjacent interstitium and inflammatory cell accumulation in adjacent airspaces.

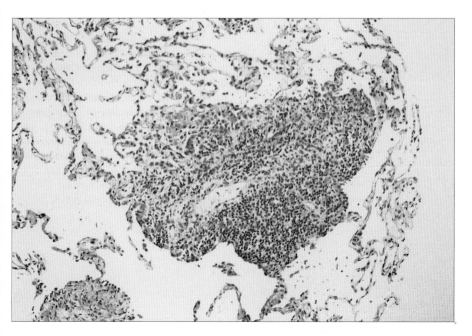

Figure 19.4
A well-circumscribed dense mononuclear cell infiltrate surrounding a vessel and showing lymphocytes adherent to endothelium at one point. The infiltrate has expanded the perivascular adventitia and begun to involve adjacent alveolar walls with intra-alveolar macrophages and inflammatory cells. These features of alveolar involvement mark the transition from A2 to A3 rejection.

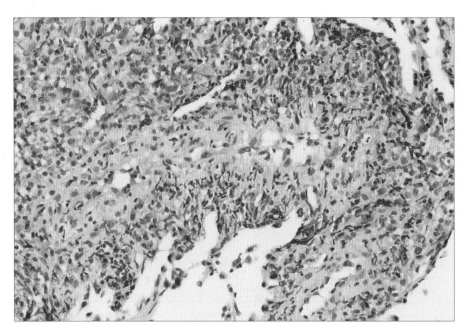

Figure 19.5
A high-power view of grade A3 rejection shows the mixed nature of the inflammatory infiltrate with small and large lymphocytes, macrophages and polymorphs. The mononuclear cells adherent to endothelium indicate endothelialitis. The airspaces contain macrophages and lymphocytes as part of the inflammatory process. The adjacent alveolar lining cells show cuboidal hyperplasia. The density of the cellular infiltrate may be less in the higher grades of rejection than in the lower grades due to edema and expansion of the perivascular space. This Grade A3 rejection shows significant numbers of polymorphs in the infiltrate. Note that these are diffuse and not forming microabscesses. (c.f. in viral alveolitis). Endothelialitis is prominent with marked endothelial cell hyperplasia and inflammatory cell infiltration.

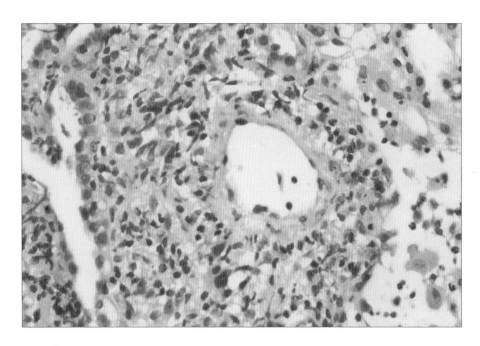

Figure 19.6
Extension of the infiltrate into adjacent alveolar walls involves cuboidal alveolar epithelial hyperplasia. The predominance of large lymphocytes in A3 rejection is well-shown. The expansion of the 'potential space' of the perivascular adventitia is also clearly visible.

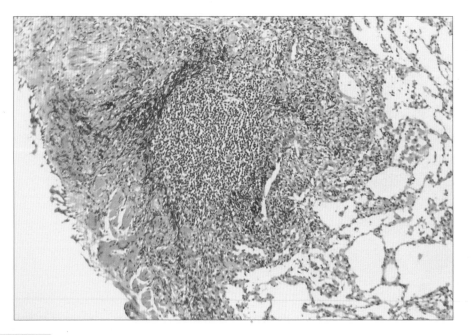

Figure 19.7
This biopsy shows perivascular infiltration with some early involvement of adjacent alveolar walls and confluence of the infiltrate with peribronchiolar infiltration with reduction of the bronchiolar lumen to a slit. The mucosal surface of the parent airway shows some epithelial loss and mild inflammatory cell infiltration with prominent bronchiolar smooth muscle. The nodular mononuclear infiltrate adjacent to the airway is suggestive of concomitant bronchus associated lymphoid tissue.

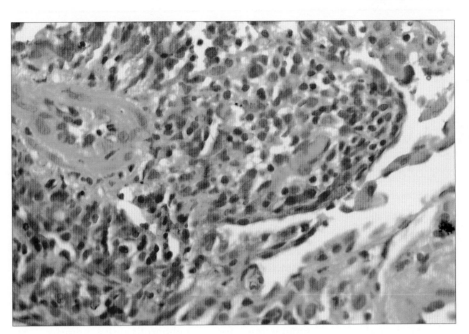

Figure 19.8
In transbronchial biopsies most of the perivascular infiltrates in rejection are seen around veins and venules. Arterioles can also be involved. This biopsy shows a perivascular infiltrate of Grade A3 severity surrounding an arteriole which shows endothelialitis.

SECTION TWENTY
GRADE A4 REJECTION
(SEVERE ACUTE REJECTION)

In Grade A4 acute rejection, the most severe grade, the cellular infiltration is diffuse with perivascular, interstitial and alveolar infiltrates. There is prominent alveolar epithelial cell damage with necrosis, hyaline membranes, hemorrhage and frequent neutrophils and macrophages. Ultimately there may be parenchymal necrosis, infarction and necrotizing vasculitis. In adequate samples the diffuse nature of this grade and the centering of the infiltrates on vessels and airways enables distinction from other causes of post-transplantation diffuse alveolar damage. Open or thoracoscopic biopsies may however be required to make this distinction in rare cases. Grade A4 acute rejection is very infrequent in patients on standard immunosuppressive therapy, but may occur in patients with poor drug absorption or decreased maintenance immunosuppression for lymphoproliferative disease, for example.

Box 21   Grade A4 (severe) acute rejection

- Diffuse infiltrates
- Alveolar damage
- Necrosis, hemorrhage
- Hyaline membranes
- Necrotizing vasculitis

Perivascular and interstitial infiltrates distinguish from reperfusion/ischemic injury

---

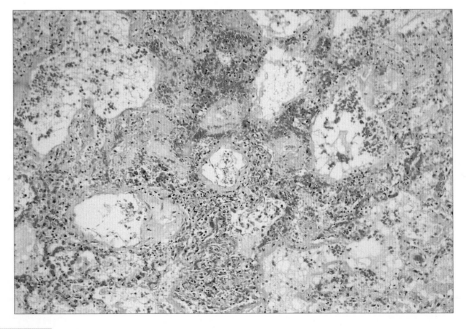

Figure 20.1
A section from an autopsy case of A4 rejection demonstrating that at scanning power the vasocentric nature of the infiltrate is clear. This is important in differentiating from non-rejection causes of diffuse alveolar damage.

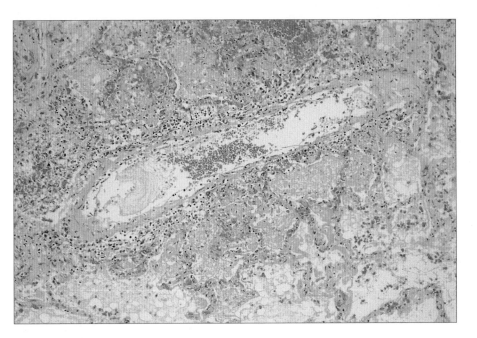

Figure 20.2
This section is also taken from autopsy lung. The perivascular infiltrate is associated with hemorrhage and edema with alveolar capillary congestion and hyaline membrane formation. We have not seen hyaline membrane formation or this degree of alveolar damage on transbronchial biopsies of A4 rejection.

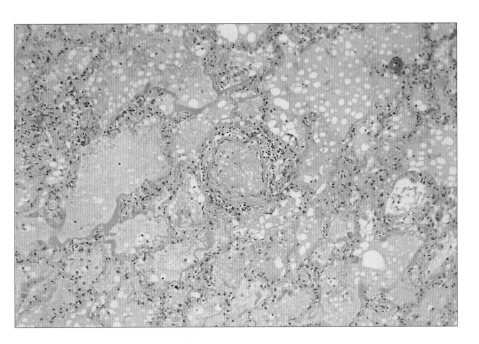

Figure 20.3
A further view of A4 rejection in the autopsy case clearly demonstrating the perivascular nature of a loose and edematous mononuclear cell infiltrate. Hyaline membranes are well-established. Perivascular distribution is not a feature of diffuse alveolar damage due to re-implantation/perfusion injury, infection, hypovolemic shock or other causes of post-transplantation diffuse alveolar damage.

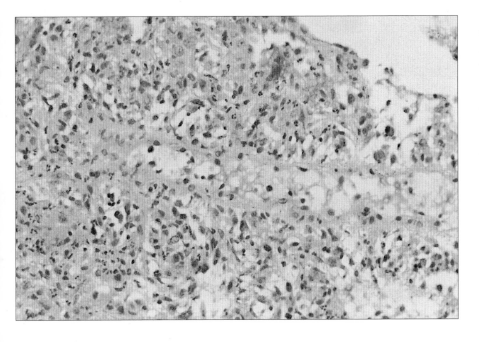

Figure 20.4
The highest grade of acute rejection is demonstrated at high-power in this transbronchial biopsy. The infiltrate is perivascular in distribution with a small proportion of small mature lymphocytes, the majority of cells being transformed lymphocytes, polymorphs, eosinophils and macrophages. Polymorphs and eosinophils are present in the endothelium indicating an active endothelialitis. The infiltrating inflammatory process is edematous, so the apparent low density of the infiltrate can be misleading at scanning magnification. This patient with cystic fibrosis had been unable to absorb adequate levels of cyclosporine due to related gastrointestinal dysfunction and developed severe acute rejection. A good response was obtained to augmented immunosuppression intravenously.

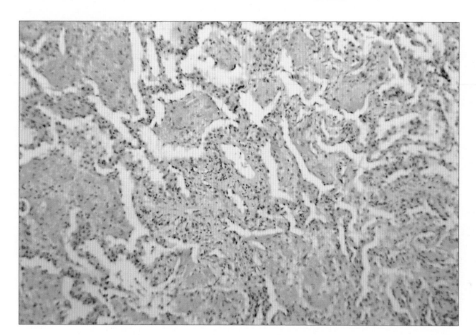

Figure 20.5
A transbronchial biopsy showing a central perivascular collection of mixed mononuclear and acute inflammatory cells with endothelialitis and extension into all adjacent alveolar walls. The airspaces contain both inflammatory cells and fibrin. No hyaline membranes are seen. The perivascular distribution of the main cellular component of this lung inflammation is clearly demonstrated.

ACUTE LUNG REJECTION INVOLVING AIRWAYS

The basis for grading acute pulmonary rejection is the presence and severity of perivascular and interstitial infiltrates in both the 1990 and 1995 Working Formulations. There is often accompanying peribronchial and peribronchiolar infiltration which can be identified in adequate transbronchial biopsies. This involvement of airways is seen more frequently in the higher grades of acute rejection. The differential diagnosis of infection is a much greater problem in the diagnosis and grading of airways rejection, but it is quite clear that in the absence of infection there is a recognizable pattern of lymphocytic bronchitis and bronchiolitis which represents acute airways rejection. The histologic features range from simple non-infiltrative mononuclear cell cuffing of the airways to mucosal infiltration with ulceration and ultimately necrosis. The 1990 classification included four suffices to indicate the presence or absence of bronchial or bronchiolar infiltrates, but did not reflect the intensity of this inflammatory process. The 1995 modification allows for grading of the airway inflammation in terms of presence and intensity, but does not distinguish large from small airway involvement. In practice the difficulty of absolutely excluding infection in the airways together with sampling problems and tangential cutting makes for considerable difficulty in applying this B grade on a day-to-day basis. It can however be applied retrospectively with the knowledge of culture and serology results and indeed studies of this type have recognized the potential for acute airways rejection to develop into obliterative bronchiolitis ie chronic airways rejection.

Examination of the concomitant bronchial aspirate or lavage is essential for the correct interpretation of airway changes. An intensely purulent aspirate is likely to represent airways infection rather than airways rejection in which macrophages and lymphocytes predominate. It is imperative that *adequate* parenchymal samples of lung tissue are available for the grading of lung rejection which is based on the A (perivascular and interstitial) grade. Grading bronchial/bronchiolar samples in less than adequate biopsies is not an adequate substitute.

The four A grades of acute rejection severity have stood the test of time in reflecting the extent of damage to the graft, its reversibility and prognosis in terms of developing chronic rejection. The A grades have also allowed the development of a treatment threshold, i.e. Grade A2 rejection and greater inevitably requiring augmented immunosuppression. This information is not as readily available for airways rejection, though in the setting of adequate biopsy fragments high-grade airways rejection in the absence of perivascular infiltrates would be an indication for augmented immunosuppression in the absence of infection.

In those centers where airway inflammation is given a numerical grade the designation of acute rejection with co-existent airway inflammation would be as follows:

Acute rejection grade A – with airways inflammation grade B – e.g. moderate acute rejection grade A3 with airways inflammation grade B3 would be designated A3, B3.

Lymphocytic bronchitis/bronchiolitis would be designated A0, B1 to 4 according to intensity. This format emphasizes the perivascular infiltrates as the main focus in the histologic classification of acute lung rejection.

Due to the limitations of bronchiolar sampling and histologic interpretation in transbronchial biopsies, some centers have studied endobronchial biopsies. These samples are not specifically addressed in the Working Formulation and are not standard samples for diagnosis. However, they form a useful adjunct and have demonstrated the stable lung transplant airway to be abnormal compared with normal subjects.

GRADE B0–B4 REJECTION

GRADE B0 REJECTION

The airways in the biopsy show no evidence of inflammation.

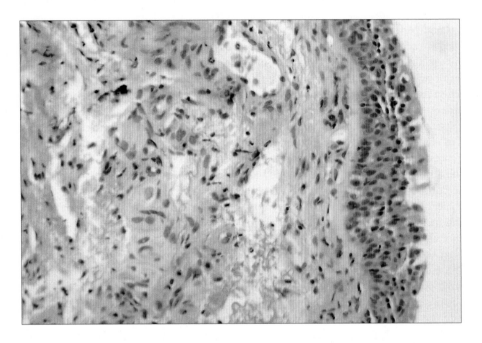

Figure 21.1
Normal airway with pseudostratified respiratory epithelium and no excess of inflammatory cells.

GRADE B1 REJECTION

Minimal airway inflammation. Scattered infrequent mature mononuclear cells are present within the submucosa of bronchi or bronchioles in this grade.

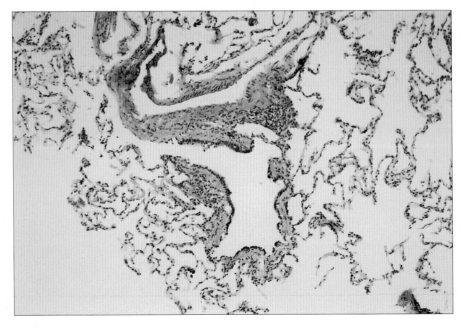

Figure 21.2
A transbronchial biopsy showing infrequent mononuclear cells in submucosa including some macrophages. The bronchiolar epithelium is intact.

GRADE B2 REJECTION

Mild airway inflammation. Cuffing of bronchioles and/or bronchi are seen with an infiltrate of mononuclear cells, some plasmacytoid and transformed with occasional eosinophils. Lymphocytes may infiltrate the epithelium, but this is not associated with epithelial damage of any kind.

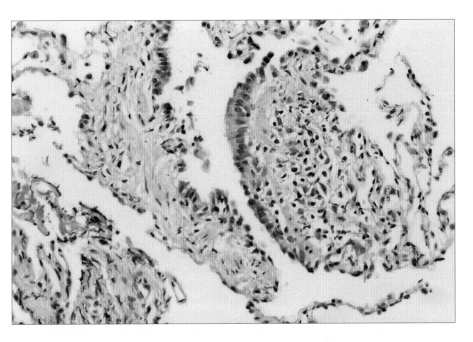

Figure 21.3

A bronchiole in a transbronchial biopsy showing intact respiratory type epithelium lining it in part with attenuated epithelium elsewhere. There is a mixed mononuclear infiltrate with small and large lymphocytes with some extension into the attenuated epithelium. The lumen of the bronchiole is free from inflammatory cells. A small amount of fibrin is noted in adjacent alveolar spaces. This was an isolated finding in the parenchyma with no evidence infection by culture or serology. This is an example of B2 airways inflammation.

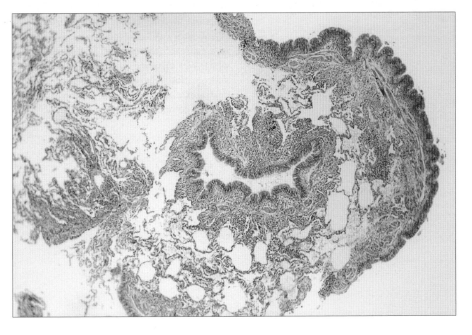

Figure 21.4

Low-power view of bronchioles in a transbronchial biopsy showing dense peribronchiolar cuffing by mononuclear cells. Even at low-power it is clear that the respiratory epithelium is intact and the lumen is free from inflammatory cells. There is no ulceration. The adjacent alveolar walls and spaces are free from involvement. This is a lymphocytic bronchiolitis consistent with acute rejection as a cause as no evidence of airways infection was found on microscopy or culture.

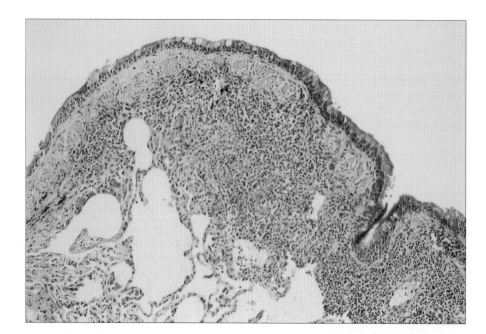

Figure 21.5

A transbronchial biopsy with a well orientated bronchiole showing cellular infiltration which is circumferential and leaves the epithelium intact. The adjacent parenchyma is free from inflammation. There was no evidence of perivascular infiltrates of acute rejection.

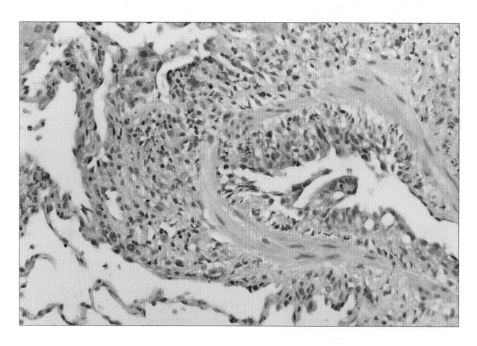

Figure 21.6

A transbronchial biopsy in which a bronchiole shows infiltration by lymphocytes, macrophages and polymorphs both in the epithelium and in the peribronchiolar adventitia. The epithelium is heavily infiltrated. The polymorphs are dispersed and are not forming microabscesses. There are hyperplastic changes in the epithelial cells together with metaplasia. There is some extension of the inflammation into peribronchiolar alveolar walls but alveolar spaces are free from inflammatory cells. Infection was excluded as a cause of inflammation in this case which was classified as B2 airways inflammation. There were mild perivascular infiltrates elsewhere in the parenchyma giving a composite grade of A2, B2.

GRADE B3 REJECTION

Moderate airway inflammation. A denser band-like infiltrate of mononuclear cells is present in the submucosa of bronchi and/or bronchioles with many more activated lymphocytes and eosinophils. The presence of lymphocytes within the epithelium itself is more marked with epithelial cell necrosis, attenuation or metaplasia. Polymorphs may be included. The epithelial surface is intact.

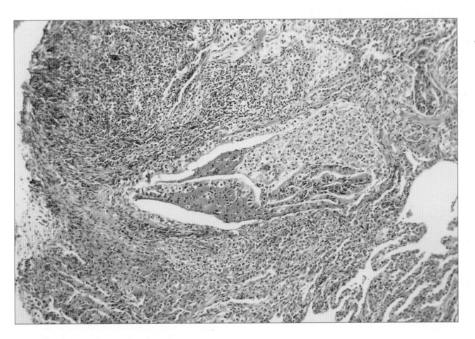

Figure 21.7

A densely infiltrated bronchiole in a transbronchial biopsy with infiltration by mononuclear cells and polymorphs and accumulation of inflammatory cells in the lumen. The epithelium is intact for the most part but heavily infiltrated by inflammatory cells. There is severe attenuation and focal ulceration in the lining of part of the bronchiole. The absence of infection allowed Grade B3 airways inflammation to be ascribed to rejection in this case. Moderate perivascular infiltrates elsewhere in the biopsy parenchyma indicated Grade A3, B3. The patient made an excellent response to augmented immunosuppression.

GRADE B4 REJECTION

Severe airway inflammation. The dense infiltrate of cells as seen in B3 is associated with epithelial damage including ulceration with fibrinopurulent exudation and epithelial cell necrosis. The infiltrates are more diffuse and in the presence of edema and hemorrhage may appear less dense than in the lower B grades.

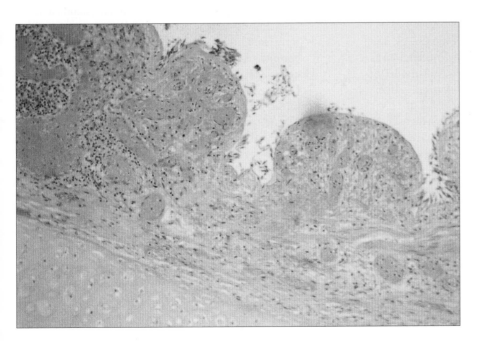

Figure 21.8

Ulcerated airway with necrosis and hemorrhage from a patient who died of acute rejection. No organisms were cultured. This B4 airways damage was associated with A4 parenchymal rejection i.e. A4, B4. B4 acute rejection is extremely rare in transbronchial biopsies as there is usually at least an element of a concomitant/ superadded infection precluding accurate grading.

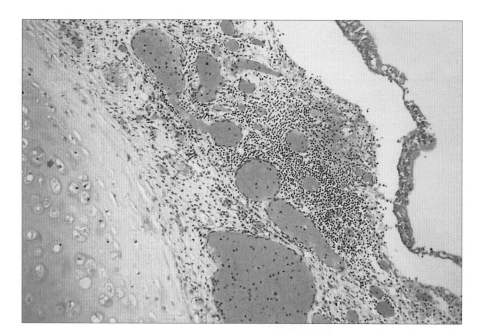

Figure 21.9
Severe acute rejection of airway with intense hemorrhage and mononuclear inflammatory cell infiltrate. There is edema and detachment of the overlying epithelium which elsewhere was ulcerated (see Figure 21.8). This intense inflammation corresponded to erythema on the donor side of the anastomosis whereas in infection there is involvement of both recipient and donor airway.

Box 22 Airway inflammation – Grade B

Lymphocytic bronchitis/bronchiolitis

B: 0–4   Grades can be assigned or presence/absence recorded

B0: Normal   B3: Moderate
B1: Minimal   B4: Severe
B2: Mild

BX: ungradeable, due to sampling problems, infection, tangential cutting

---

Box 23 Causes of acute bronchitis/bronchiolitis in the lung transplant recipient

1.   Reperfusion injury with diffuse alveolar damage
2.   Acute cellular rejection (B1–4)
3.   Obliterative bronchiolitis (Ca)
4.   Infection
5.   Aspiration
6.   Recurrent disease
7.   Others

FURTHER READING

Boehler A, Chamberlain D, Kesten S, Slutsky AS, Liu M, Keshavjee S. Lymphocytic airway infiltration as a precursor to fibrous obliteration in a rat model of bronchiolitis obliterans. *Transplantation* 1997; 64;311–7.

Fournier M, Igual J, Groussard O *et al*. Mucosal T-lymphocytes in central airways of lung transplant recipients. *Am J Respir Crit Care Med* 1995; 151:1974–80.

Fournier M, Lebargy F, Ladurie FLR, Lenormand E, Pariente R. Intraepithelial T-lymphocyte subsets in the airways of normal subjects and of patients with chronic bronchitis. *Am Rev Resp Dis* 1989; 140:737–42.

Glanville AR, Tazelaar HD, Theodore J *et al*. The distribution of MHC class I and class II antigens on bronchial epithelium. *Am Rev Resp Dis* 1989; 139:330–4.

Hasegawa T, Iacono A, Yousem SA. The significance of bronchus-associated lymphoid tissue in human lung transplantation: is there an association with acute and chronic rejection? *Transplantation* 1999;15:381–5.

Hruban RH, Beschorner WE, Baumgartner WA *et al*. Diagnosis of lung allograft rejection by bronchial intraepithelial Leu-7 positive T-lymphocytes. *J Thorac Cardiovasc Surg* 1988;96:939–46.

Hruban RH, Beschorner WE, Hutchins GM. Lymphocytic bronchitis and lung allograft rejection. *Transplantation* 1990;50:723.

Liakakos P, Snell GI, Ward C *et al*. Bronchial hyperresponsiveness in lung transplant recipients: lack of correlation with airway inflammation. *Thorax* 1997;52:551–6.

O'Shaughnessy TC, Ansari TW, Barnes NC, Jeffery PK. Inflammation in bronchial biopsies of subjects with chronic bronchitis: inverse relationship of CD8+ T lymphocytes with FEV_1. *Am J Respir Crit Care Med* 1997;155:852–7.

Ohori NP, Iacono AT, Grgurich WF, Yousem SA. Significance of acute bronchiolitis/bronchiolitis in the lung transplant recipient. *Am J Surg Pathol* 1994; **18**:1192–1204.

Pabst R. Is BALT a major component of the human lung immune system? *Immunol Today* 1992;**13**:119–121.

Ross DJ, Markevski A, Kramer M, Kass RM. 'Refractoriness' of airflow obstruction associated with isolated lymphocytic bronchiolitis/bronchitis in pulmonary allografts. *J Heart Lung Transplant* 1998;**16**:832–8.

Snell GI, Ward C, Wilson JW, Orsida B, Williams TJ, Walters EH. Immunopathological changes in the airways of stable lung transplant recipients. *Thorax* 1997;**52**:322–8.

Ward C, Snell GI, Zheng L *et al*. Endobronchial biopsy and bronchoalveolar lavage in stable lung transplant recipients in chronic rejection. *Am J Respir Crit Car Med* 1998;**158**:84–91.

Yousem SA, Dauber JH, Griffith BP. Bronchial cartilage alterations in lung transplantation. *Chest* 1990; **98**:1121–24.

Yousem SA, Paradis IL, Dauber JA *et al*. Large airway inflammation in heart–lung recipients – its significance and prognostic implications. *Transplantation* 1990;**49**:654.

Yousem SA. Lymphocytic bronchitis/bronchiolitis in lung allograft recipients. *Am J Surg Pathol* 1993;**17**:491–6.

SECTION TWENTY-TWO

GRADE C CHRONIC AIRWAY REJECTION – OBLITERATIVE BRONCHIOLITIS

Obliterative bronchiolitis (bronchiolitis obliterans) is a fibroproliferative scarring disorder of membranous and respiratory bronchioles which is the morphologic hallmark of chronic airway rejection in the transplanted lung. The scar tissue involving bronchioles consists of dense eosinophilic hyaline fibrous submucosal plaques resulting in partial or complete narrowing of the airway lumen. It can be concentric or eccentric and may extend into the wall with fragmentation and destruction of elastica and smooth muscle reaching peribronchiolar adventitia. The epithelial lining may remain of respiratory ciliated type but often undergoes squamous metaplasia and attenuation. The epithelium is also frequently infiltrated by acute inflammatory cells as the presence of chronic airways rejection predisposes to airways infection. Foamy macrophages are present both within the lumen of the affected bronchiole and distally in airspaces due to mucostasis. The foamy cells may also become incorporated into the fibrous scar as an integral part of the lesion of obliterative bronchiolitis.

The diagnosis of obliterative bronchiolitis is often a combination of clinical and pathologic criteria. The patients can be classified as having bronchiolitis obliterans syndrome (BOS) with breathlessness, cough and a decline in their spirometry. This can be Grade 1 to 3 according to severity (Table 5). This clinical classification notes whether or not there is histologic confirmation of the obliterative bronchiolitis on transbronchial biopsy material. Transbronchial biopsies are a relatively insensitive method of diagnosing obliterative bronchiolitis due to the patchy nature of the disease particularly in its early stages and the paucity of bronchioles

in many biopsies. The diagnostic yield can however be enhanced by increasing the number of biopsy fragments taken, the amount of tissue examined by serial sections and the use of connective tissue stains to diagnose subtle submucosal fibrosis which would otherwise be overlooked.

Transbronchial biopsies are usually performed in the setting of irreversible decline in lung function (BOS) to exclude treatable causes such as acute rejection or infection rather than to obtain tissue to confirm obliterative bronchiolitis histologically.

Obliterative bronchiolitis must be distinguished from organizing pneumonia and bronchiolitis obliterans organizing pneumonia (BOOP) where there is *intra-alveolar* fibroproliferation in the form of granulation tissue plugs. The obliterative bronchiolitis of chronic airways rejection is exquisitely confined to the airways without involvement of alveolar spaces. Any alveolar involvement is due to organization of other pathologic processes including infection, acute rejection, aspiration and diffuse alveolar damage and is designated organizing pneumonia.

In the active form of obliterative bronchiolitis there is mononuclear cell infiltration of airways including peribronchiolar tissue, usually with epithelial damage and intrabronchiolar inflammation. This is in addition to the submucosal fibrosis which defines the lesion.

In the inactive form of obliterative bronchiolitis, dense fibrous scarring is seen without cellular infiltrates. This is interpreted as representing a more mature lesion with less likelihood of response to augmented immunosuppression. In the 1990 Working Formulation obliterative bronchiolitis was divided into subtotal and total forms which proved to be difficult to assess on transbronchial biopsy material and added nothing further to the BOS diagnosis by this distinction. Therefore in the 1995 Working Formulation obliterative bronchiolitis is simply graded as active versus inactive, i.e. Grade Ca or Cb.

Bronchi may be obliterated in chronic rejection i.e. obliterative bronchitis and large airways show bronchiectasis. Bronchial dilatation has been shown to be a useful CT feature of obliterative bronchiolitis.

Table 5
BOS classification using Fev$_1$ values

Stage	FEV$_1$ values, % of post-transplant baseline	Severity of BOS
0	>80	No significant abnormality
I	66–80	Mild BOS
2	51–65	Moderate BOS
3	≤50	Severe BOS

From: Cooper *et al. J Heart Lung Transplant* 1993;**12**:713–16.

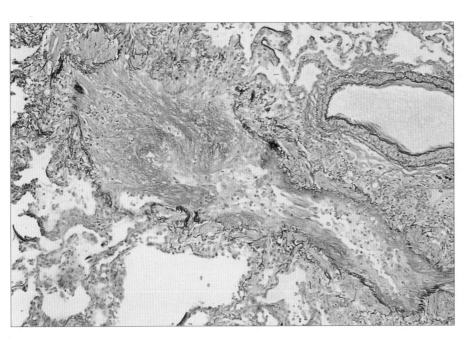

Figure 22.1
Open lung biopsy with bronchiole eccentrically occluded by fibrous tissue with foamy macrophages within the residual bronchiolar lumen. There is no active inflammatory infiltrate. Note the accompanying arterial vessel is unremarkable. Elastic van Gieson stain. Obliterative bronchiolitis should always be assessed with a routine connective tissue stain.

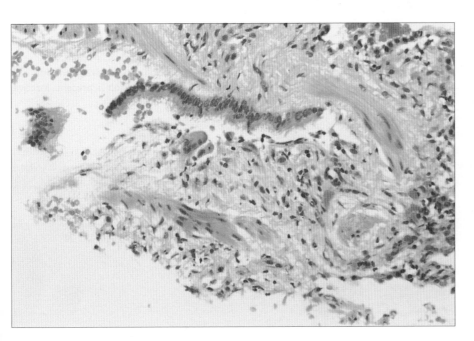

Figure 22.2
A transbronchial biopsy showing a bronchiole with partial respiratory epithelial lining and clearly defined smooth muscle in its wall. There is eccentric cellular fibroproliferative tissue significantly reducing the lumen. There is also a mild degree of inflammation external to the adventitia. A single giant cell is noted on the surface of the occluding scar tissue raising the possibility of aspiration.

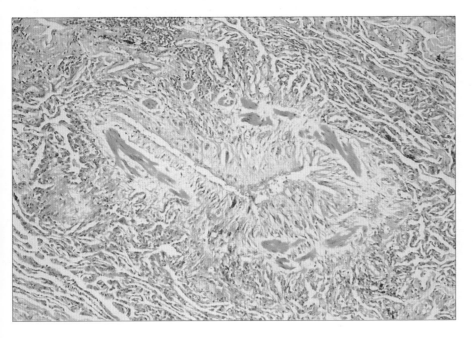

Figure 22.3
Open lung biopsy from a patient whose immunosuppression was reduced during treatment of lymphoproliferative disease. Established obliterative bronchiolitis is present with little cellular infiltrate and marked concentric fibrotic narrowing of the bronchiolar lumen. Attenuated respiratory epithelium remains. The smooth muscle in the wall is interrupted by the bronchiolar fibrosis.

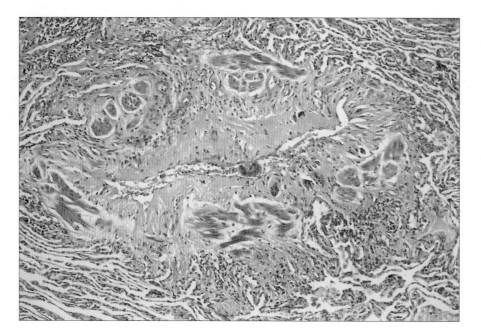

Figure 22.4
Another bronchiole from the same open lung biopsy showing obliterative bronchiolitis with giant cells on the surface of the fibrous tissue. This is a not uncommon finding, again raising the possibility of aspiration which is clinically underestimated in lung transplant recipients. Non-immune causes such as aspiration may accelerate obliterative bronchiolitis when superimposed on immune factors.

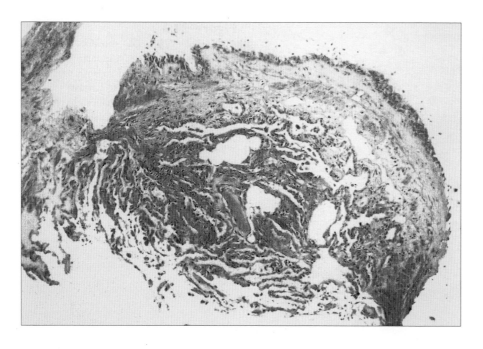

Figure 22.5
Transbronchial biopsy showing acellular fibrous plaque beneath epithelium with some attenuation of underlying smooth muscle. No inflammation is present. Inactive obliterative bronchiolitis.

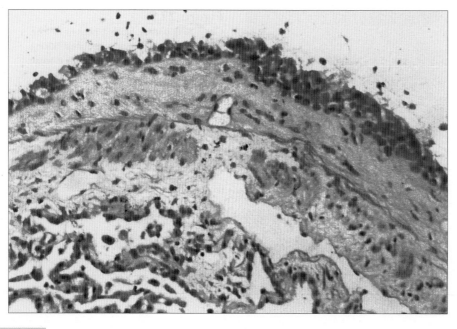

Figure 22.6
Higher power view showing acellular subepithelial fibrosis of early obliterative bronchiolitis. This can be easily overlooked at low-power.

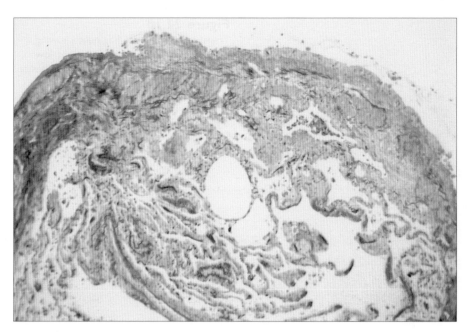

Figure 22.7
Elastic van Gieson staining highlights the dense abnormal fibrous tissue even at low-power in the transbronchial biopsy shown in Figs. 22.5 and 22.6.

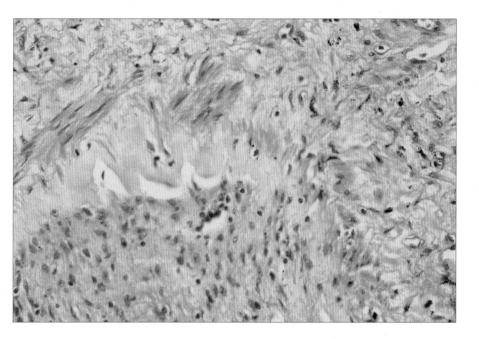

Figure 22.8
High-power of obliterative bronchiolitis with dense acellular fibrosis superimposed on which there is cellular fibroproliferative occluding the lumen. Fragments of residual mural smooth muscle are seen external to the fibrous plaque. This morphologic appearance suggests that, in some airways at least, occlusion is due to a 'two-hit' process and supports a multifactorial etiology in which rejection is a major factor.

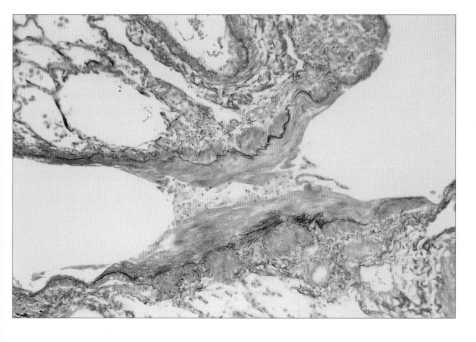

Figure 22.9
Obliterative bronchiolitis demonstrated longitudinally with reduction in lumen due to acellular hyaline fibrous plaques associated with and incorporating foamy macrophages. The lesion clearly demonstrates the restriction to airflow and its incidence is likely to be underestimated by sampling problems. Elastic van Gieson stain.

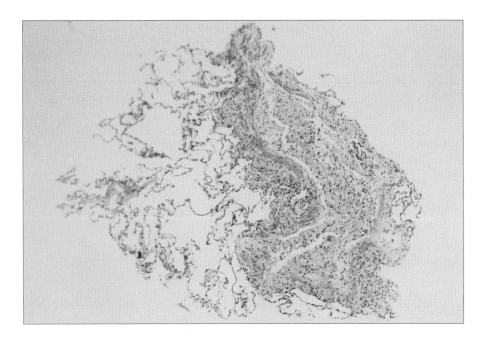

Figure 22.10
Transbronchial biopsy fragment showing a well-orientated bronchiole which at low-power shows almost total luminal occlusion.

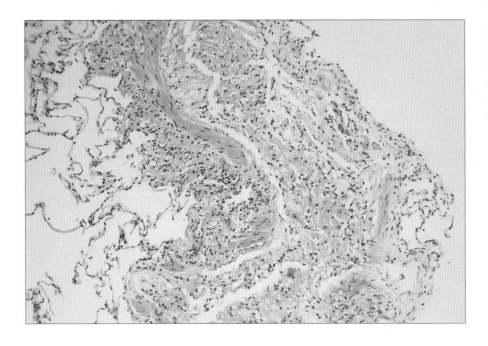

Figure 22.11
Higher power of this occluded bronchiole shows fibrous tissue with abundant macrophages and a single giant cell. Obliterative bronchiolitis, confidently diagnosed on transbronchial biopsy in a patient with irreversible decline in lung function.

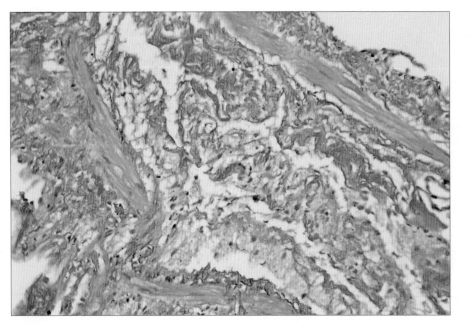

Figure 22.12
Connective tissue stain highlights the admixture of collagen and macrophages occluding the bronchiolar lumen in obliterative bronchiolitis. Foamy macrophages in distal parenchyma of a biopsy are strongly suggestive of obliteration due to bronchiolitis obliterans but may also be an integral part of the stenosing lesion as illustrated here. Elastic van Gieson stain.

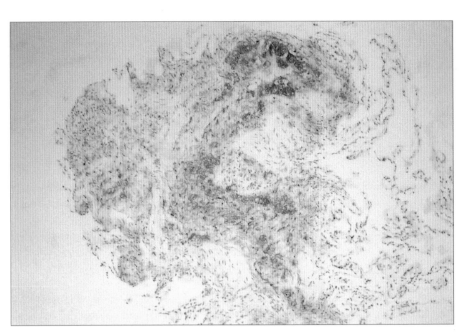

Figure 22.13
CD68 macrophage marker demonstrates the significant number of macrophages in this lesion of obliterative bronchiolitis.

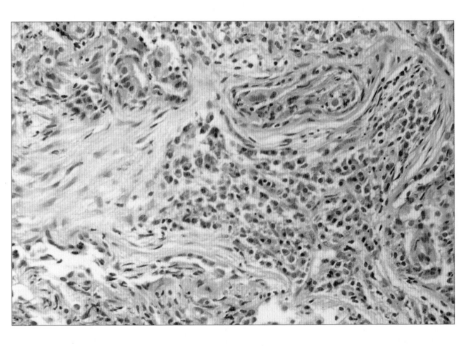

Figure 22.14
Transbronchial biopsy of organizing pneumonia with central plasma cells and other mononuclear cells in the fibrous tissue which fills alveolar spaces. This is to be contrasted with the obliterative bronchiolitis shown in other figures.

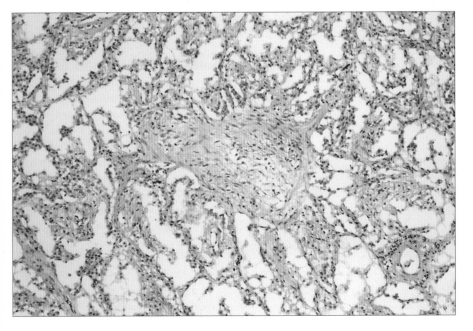

Figure 22.15
Open biopsy showing organizing pneumonia with extension into a small bronchiole. Co-existence of these two processes is common and can be extremely difficult to differentiate on small biopsy material. It is important not to confuse bronchiolitis obliterans organizing pneumonia with obliterative bronchiolitis as the clinical implications of the diagnoses are very different.

Box 25 Obliterative bronchiolitis – etiology

Evidence for chronic rejection i.e. immune

1. Severe and persistent biopsy proven acute rejection
2. Airways inflammation acute rejection
3. Association with chronic vascular rejection
4. Increased class II antigen expression
5. Leu-7+ve T-cells in bronchial epithelium in OB patients
6. Increased dendritic cells in epithelium of OB patients
7. Positive primed lymphocyte testing studies
8. CD8 +ve cells in TBB and BAL

Box 26 Obliterative bronchiolitis – etiology

Non-immune mechanisms

- Infection: Viral including CMV, RSV, adenovirus mycoplasma, chlamydia
- Ischemia, particularly chronic
- Aspiration
- Denervation
- Drugs

Box 27 Chronic airway rejection – Obliterative bronchiolitis Grade C

1. *Active* Intra and/or peribronchiolar submucosal and mural infiltrates
2. *Inactive* No cellular infiltrates

1990 categories of C1, subtotal and C2, total occlusion abolished

FURTHER READING

Abernathy EC, Hruban RH, Baumgartner WA, Reitz BA, Hutchins GM. The two forms of bronchiolitis obliterans in heart-lung transplant recipients. *Hum Pathol* 1991;**22**:1102–1110.

Al-Dossari GA, Jessurun J, Bolman RM *et al.* Pathogenesis of obliterative bronchiolitis. *Transplantation* 1995;**59**:143–5.

Boehler A, Kesten S, Weder W, Speich R. Bronchiolitis obliterans after lung transplantation. *Chest* 1998;**114**:1411–26.

Bolman RM III. Advantage – FK 506: Reduced chronic rejection for lung transplant recipients. *Ann Thorac Surg* 1995;**60**:495–6.

Burke CM, Glanville AR, Theodore J, Robin ED. Lung immunogenicity, rejection and obliterative bronchiolitis. *Chest* 1987;**92**:547–9.

Burke CM, Theodore J, Dawkins KD *et al.* Post-transplant obliterative bronchiolitis and other late lung sequelae in human heart-lung transplantation. *Chest* 1984;**86**:824–9.

Burke CM, Yousem SA, Corris PA. Heart–lung transplantation. In: *Diseases of the bronchioles*, Chapter 17. (Ed GR Epler). Raven Press, New York, 1994; pp. 259–74.

Cagle PT, Brown RW, Frost A, Kellar C, Yousem SA. Diagnosis of chronic lung transplant rejection by transbronchial biopsy. *Modern Pathol* 1995; **8**:137–42.

Cohen M, Sahn SA. Bronchiectasis in systemic diseases. *Chest* 1999;**116**:1063–74.

Colby TV. Bronchiolar pathology. In: *Diseases of the bronchioles*. (Ed GR Epler). Raven Press, New York, 1994; pp. 77–100.

Coultas DB, Funk LM. Postinfectious bronchiolitis obliterans. In: *Diseases of the Bronchioles*, Chapter 13. (Ed GR Epler). Raven Press, New York 1994; pp. 215–29.

El-Gamel A, Sim E, Hasleton P *et al.* Transforming growth factor beta (TGF-β) and obliterative bronchiolitis following pulmonary transplantation. *J Heart Lung Transplant* 1999;**18**:828–37.

Epler GR, Colby TV. The spectrum of bronchiolitis obliterans. *Chest* 1983;**83**:161–2.

Frost AE, Keller CA, Cagle PT. Severe ischaemic injury to the proximal airway following lung transplantation. Immediate and long-term effects on bronchial cartilage. *Chest* 1993;**103**:1899–1901.

Girgis RE, Tu I, Berry GJ *et al.* Risk factors for the development of obliterative bronchiolitis after lung transplantation. *J Heart Lung Transplant* 1996; **15**:1200–8.

Glanville AR, Baldwin JC, Burke CM, Theodore J, Robin ED. Obliterative bronchiolitis after heart–lung transplantation: apparent arrest by augmented immunosuppression. *Ann Intern Med* 1987; **107**:300–4.

Hirsch J, Elssner A, Mazur G *et al.* Bronchiolitis obliterans syndrome after (heart–) lung transplantation. Impaired antiprotease defence and increased oxidant activity. *Am J Respir Crit Care Med* 1999; **160**:1640–6.

Keller CA, Cagle PT, Brown RW, Noon G, Frost AE. Bronchiolitis obliterans in recipients of single, double and heart–lung transplantation. *Chest* 1995; **107**:973–80.

Lentz D, Bergin CJ, Berry G J, Stoehr C, Theodore J. Diagnosis of bronchiolitis obilterans in heart–lung transplantation patients: Importance of bronchial dilatation on CT. *AJR* 1992;**159**:463–7.

Levine SM, Bryan CL. Bronchiolitis obliterans in lung transplant recipients. *Chest* 1995;**107**:894–6.

Mauck KA, Hosenpud JD. The bronchial epithelium: A potential allogeneic target for chronic rejection after lung transplantation. *J Heart Lung Transplant* 1996;**15**:709–14.

Maurer JR. Lung transplantation bronchiolitis obliterans. In: *Diseases of the bronchioles*, Chapter 18. (Ed GR Epler). Raven Press, New York, 1994; pp.275–89.

Milne DS, Gascoigne A, Wilkes J *et al.* The immuno-histopathology of obliterative bronchiolitis following lung transplantation. *Transplantation* 1992;**54**:748–50.

Nathan SD, Ross DJ, Belman MJ. *et al.* Bronchiolitis obliterans in single-lung transplant recipients. *Chest* 1995;**107**:967–72.

Novick RJ, Schäfers H-J, Stitt L *et al.* Cardiac and pulmonary replacement. Recurrence of obliterative bronchiolitis and determinants of outcome in 139 pulmonary retransplant recipients. *J Thorac Cardiovasc Surg* 1995;**110**:1402–14.

Paradis IL, Yousem SA, Griffith B. Airway obstruction and bronchiolitis obliterans after lung transplantation. *Clin Chest Med* 1993;**14**:751–63.

Philit F, Wiesendanger T, Archimbaud E, Mornex J-F, Brune J, Cordier J-F. Post-transplant obstructive lung disease ('bronchiolitis obliterans'): a clinical comparative study of bone marrow and lung transplant patients. *Eur Respir J* 1995;**8**:551–8.

Reichenspurner H, Girgis RE, Robbins RC *et al.* Stanford experience with obliterative bronchiolitis after lung and heart lung transplantation. *Ann Thorac Surg* 1996;**62**:1467–73.

Reinsmoen NL, Bolman RM, Savik K, Butters K, Hertz MI. Are multiple immunopathogenetic events occurring during the development of obliterative bronchiolitis and acute rejection?. *Transplantation* 1993;**55**:1040–44.

Riise GC, Williams A, Kjellström C, Schersten H, Andersson BA, Kelly FJ. Bronchiolitis obliterans syndrome in lung transplant recipients is associated with increased neutrophil activity and decreased antioxidant status in the lung. *Eur Respir J* 1998;**12**:82–8.

Schlesinger C, Neyer C A, Veeraraghavan S, Koss MN. Constrictive (obliterative) bronchiolitis: diagnosis, etiology, and a critical review of the literature. *Ann Diagn Pathol* 1998;**2**:321–34.

Scott JP, Higenbottam TW, Clelland CA *et al.* Natural history of chronic rejection in heart–lung transplant recipients. *J Heart Transplant* 1990;**9**:510–15.

Scott JP, Higenbottam TW, Sharples L *et al.* Risk factors of obliterative bronchiolitis in heart–lung transplant recipients. *Transplantation* 1991;**51**:813–17.

Sharples LD, Tamm M, McNeil K *et al.* Development of bronchiolitis obliterans syndrome in recipients of heart–lung transplantation: early risk factors. *Transplantation* 1996;**61**:560–66.

Sharples L, Scott J, Dennis C *et al.* Risk factors for survival following combined heart–lung transplantation. *Transplantation* 1994;**57**:218–23.

Skeens JL, Fuhrman CR, Yousem SA. Bronchiolitis obliterans in heart-lung transplantation patients: Radiological findings in 11 patients. *AJR* 1989;**153**:253–6.

Smith MA, Sundaresan S, Mohanakumar T *et al.* Effect of development of antibodies to HLA and cytomegalovirus mismatch on lung transplantation survival and development of bronchiolitis obliterans syndrome. *J Thorac Cardiovasc Surg* 1998;**116**:812–20.

Snell GI, Ward C, Wilson JW, Orsida B, Williams TJ, Walter EH. Immunopathological changes in the airways of stable lung transplant recipients. *Thorax* 1997; **52**:322–8.

Sundaresan S, Trulock EP, Mohanakumar T, Cooper JD, Patterson A, The Washington University Lung Transplant Group. Prevalence and outcome of bronchiolitis obliterans syndrome after lung transplantation. *Ann Thorac Surg* 1995;**60**:1341–7.

Tazelaar HD, Yousem SA. The pathology of combined heart-lung transplantation. An autopsy study. *Hum Pathol* 1988;**119**:1403–16.

Tullius SG, Tilney NL. Both alloantigen-dependent and -independent factors influence chronic allograft rejection. *Transplantation* 1995;**3**:313–18.

Yousem SA, Dauber JA, Keenan R, Paradis IL, Zeevi A, Griffith BP. Does histologic acute rejection in lung allografts predict the development of bronchiolitis obliterans? *Transplantation* 1991;**52**:306–9.

Yousem SA, Isaacs A. Pulmonary neuroendocrine cells in the airways of lung allografts. *Transplantation* 1995;**59**:1070–73.

Yousem SA, Paradis I, Griffith BP. Can transbronchial biopsy aid in the diagnosis of bronchiolitis obliterans in lung transplant recipients. *Transplantation* 1994;**57**:151–3.

Yousem SA, Suncan SR, Ohori P, Sonmez-Alpan E. Architectural remodelling of lung allografts in acute and chronic rejection. *Arch Pathol Lab Med* 1992;**116**:1175–80.

Yousem SA. Small airway injury in heart-lung transplant recipients. *Semin Respir Med* 1992;**13**:85–93

Zheng L, Orsida BE, Ward C *et al.* Airway vascular changes in lung allograft recipients. *J Heart Lung Transplant* 1999;**18**:231–8.

Zheng L, Ward C, Snell GI. Scar collagen deposition in the airways of allografts of lung transplant recipients. *Am J Respir Crit Care Med* 1997;**155**:2072–77.

GRADE D CHRONIC VASCULAR REJECTION

Chronic vascular rejection in the lung consists of fibrointimal thickening of arteries and veins similar to that seen in the vessels of the transplanted heart in chronic rejection. There may be an active component with subendothelial intimal and/or medial mononuclear cell infiltrates as in other solid organ chronic rejection. However in the lung the most common appearance is of rather acellular fibrointimal thickening particularly involving veins. The clinical significance of these pathologic changes is uncertain but it is noted to correlate with the presence of coronary artery disease in combined heart–lung allografts and also with obliterative bronchiolitis in lung allografts. As well as being a manifestation of chronic rejection these non-specific pulmonary vascular changes could also include reaction to preservation/ischemic injury, parenchymal scarring and thrombosis/embolism. They are easily seen in transbronchial biopsies and occur surprisingly early after grafting implying that these other causes are important and care should be taken not to overdiagnose chronic vascular rejection.

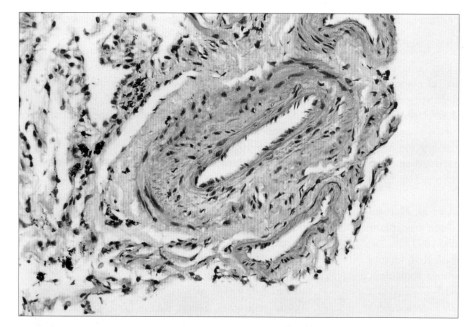

Figure 23.1
Transbronchial biopsy showing a thickened vessel with fibrointimal fibrosis and little inflammatory cell infiltrate.

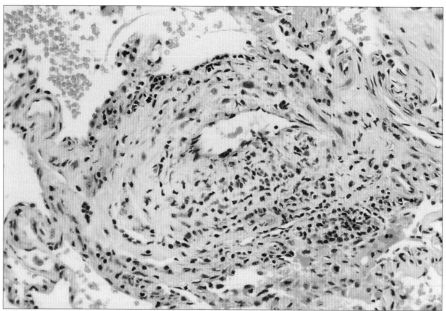

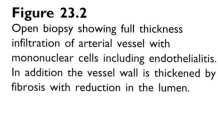

Figure 23.2
Open biopsy showing full thickness infiltration of arterial vessel with mononuclear cells including endothelialitis. In addition the vessel wall is thickened by fibrosis with reduction in the lumen.

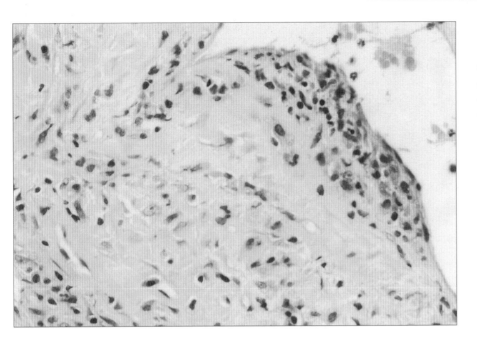

Figure 23.3
Higher power of endothelialitis (or intimitis) in vessel showing chronic vascular rejection. There is diffuse fibrosis through the vascular wall with a intense mononuclear infiltrate in the endothelium. The presence of fibrosis is the key to differentiating this lesion Grade D from acute rejection, Grade A.

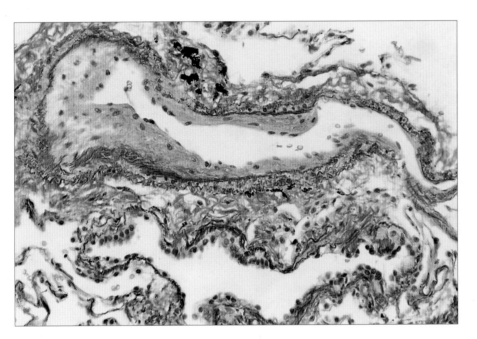

Figure 23.4
Transbronchial biopsy showing asymmetrical poorly cellular fibrosis in the intima of an arteriole. There is no significant inflammation. The accompanying bronchiole is unremarkable. In transbronchial biopsy samples vascular abnormalities are more readily seen than bronchiolar ones which is partly due to sampling and partly due to the complete lack of specificity of this type of vascular sclerosis.

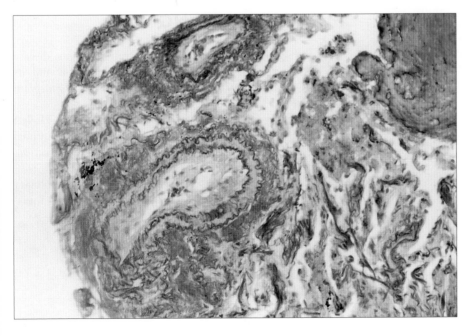

Figure 23.5
Transbronchial biopsy showing two vessels with intimal fibrosis and thickened media with muscularization. There is some increase in adventitial fibrosis. This lesion is non-specific, but is seen in this case in association with obliterative bronchiolitis in a patient with clinical bronchiolitis obliterans syndrome.

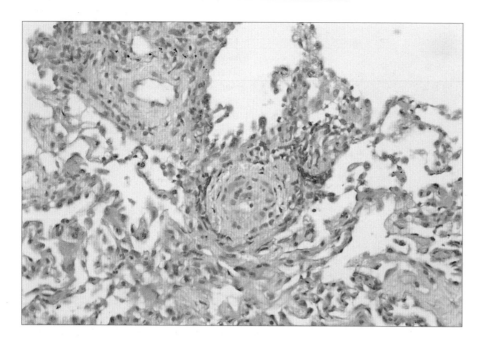

Figure 23.6
Transbronchial biopsy showing thickening of the wall of a small arteriole with endovasculitis. This is in keeping with chronic vascular rejection because of the fibrosis. A minor perivascular infiltrate is also seen i.e. A1, D.

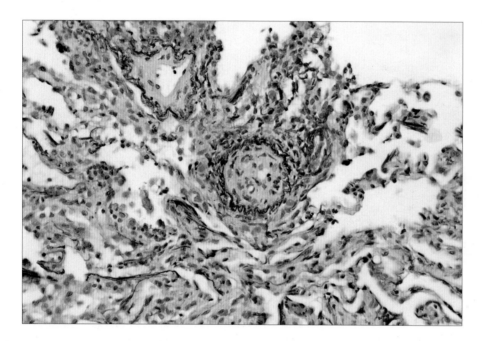

Figure 23.7
Elastic van Gieson staining of the same vessel confirms the fibrosis within the vessel wall and lumen.

Box 28 Grade D – chronic vascular rejection

- Fibrointimal proliferation of veins and arteries
- May be active mononuclear cell infiltration

FURTHER READING

Billingham ME. Pathology of graft vascular disease after heart and heart–lung transplantation and its relationship to obliterative bronchiolitis. *Transplant Proc* 1995;27:2013–16.

Geraghty JG, Stoltenbert RL, Sollinger HW, Hullett DA. Vascular smooth muscle cells and neointimal hyperplasia in chronic transplant rejection. *Transplantation* 1996;62:502–9.

Yousem SA, Paradis IL, Dauber JH *et al*. Pulmonary arteriosclerosis in long-term human heart-lung transplant recipients. *Transplantation* 1989;47:564–9.

OPPORTUNISTIC INFECTION IN THE TRANSPLANTED LUNG

Infection is the most common differential diagnosis of acute rejection and often requires biopsy and lavage. Some histologic features are identified with particular organisms, but there are also general features which are strongly suggestive of an infective process either opportunistic or common which must be recognized (Table 6). The commonest non-specific feature is a polymorphonuclear infiltrate.

Table 6
Histologic features of infection and likely organisms

Features	Organism
Perivascular infiltrates	Many
Polymorphs	Many
Perivascular edema	CMV
Endothelialitis	CMV, PCP
Eosinophils	Pseudomonas, fungus
Granulomas	PCP, fungus, TB, atypical mycobacteria
Necrosis	TB, atypical mycobacteria, HSV, fungus, PTLPD
Lymphoproliferative	EBV
Bronchitis	Bacteria, fungus, HSV, PTLPD
Bronchiolitis	Bacteria, fungus, HSV, RSV, adenovirus

Patients with lung grafts are very susceptible to common bacterial and viral infections and also to opportunistic infections. Diagnosis and treatment of these infections is a major indication for transbronchial biopsy and lavage of the post-transplant lung. Transbronchial biopsies are important in the diagnosis of CMV, *Pneumocystis carinii* and mycobacterial infections as well as *Aspergillus* infections. The accompanying lavages are often more helpful than the biopsy in the diagnosis of *Aspergillus*, *Candida* and Herpes simplex.

Special stains are mandatory in the assessment of transbronchial biopsies for opportunistic infection and the appearances should always be correlated with any accompanying lavage, culture and serologic results. The histopathology of opportunistic infection in the transplanted lung has been modified by the use of effective prophylaxis particularly against CMV and *Pneumocystis*. The florid cytomegalovirus and *Pneumocystis carinii* pneumonias seen early in the development of clinical lung transplantation are now relatively uncommon and the biopsy changes may be subtle and easily overlooked by the reporting pathologist. Examples of infections unmodified by prophylaxis are included in order to demonstrate the important diagnostic features.

The incidence of infection is greatest after augmented immunosuppression and also when obliterative bronchiolitis is established, often with large airway dilatation. Viral infections can predispose to bacterial superinfection. Infection may draw clinical attention to previously silent obliterative bronchiolitis.

Transbronchial biopsy material may not be necessary to diagnose upper airway infection. Sputum examination and culture with or without bronchoschopy and aspiration may be sufficient. Viral and fungal infections have the highest mortality but bacterial infections are most common, particularly of Gram-negative type.

The high incidence of infection is related obviously to immunosuppression but also to diminished mucociliary clearance, denervation, loss of cough reflex and the role of the graft as foreign host to infecting agents. The depletion of bronchus-associated lymphoid tissue may also be a factor in the graft, further reducing host defenses. The remaining native lung in single lung transplants may increase the risk of infection and this should be considered at the time of listing for lung transplantation. Bilateral suppurative lung disease requires that both diseased lung are removed and replaced.

Box 29 Features of infection in transbronchial biopsies

PCP may mimic rejection
Infection suggested by:
- Abundant neutrophils
- Eosinophilic infiltrate
- Granulomas
- Punctate necrosis

As with heart transplantation, CMV may be a primary infection or a reactivation. Cytomegalovirus may be a systemic infection or confined to the lungs. Where the virus is causing lung damage it is designated CMV pneumonitis, but it has to be remembered that in the immunosuppressed seropositive patient CMV infection without inflammation may be seen in biopsy material not requiring specific antiviral treatment. Monitoring of CMV antigenemia and polymerase chain reactions (PCR) is useful for assessing the significance of CMV where pneumonitis is not present on biopsy fragments. Multidisciplinary assessment is very important in determining of clinical significance.

Transbronchial biopsies from patients with unmodified CMV pneumonitis show typical features of viral alveolitis often with diffuse alveolar damage. There are prominent polymorphs in the interstitial infiltrates which may form microabscesses. Collections of polymorphs like this are not seen in acute rejection and are a useful pointer to infection, usually viral. The interstitium also appears edematous and hemorrhagic. There is perivascular edema in contrast to the mononuclear cell cuffing of acute rejection and no evidence of endothelialitis unless CMV infected endothelial cells are present in the section which is extremely rare (Table 7). Alveolar epithelial cells show marked reactive changes often with ulceration. Diagnostic intranuclear 'owl's eye' inclusions together with granular intracytoplasmic inclusions enable a firm diagnosis of CMV pneumonitis to be made. These inclusions are present in both epithelial and endothelial cells and macrophages but do not involve airways. Immunohistochemical staining for CMV can be performed but often does not add anything

further to the H & E diagnosis. The features of viral alveolitis may be present in the absence of diagnostic inclusions and in the appropriate clinical setting a diagnosis of 'preinclusion' CMV pneumonitis can be offered and treatment commenced.

Ganciclovir prophylaxis has modified the biopsy appearances of CMV pneumonitis to a focal neutrophilic pneumonitis with sparse inclusions which may require the examination of multiple serial sections. The infected cells often do not show the characteristic cytomegaly and the intranuclear inclusions may be eosinophilic and degenerate in appearance. In this setting immunohistochemical staining for CMV may be more helpful. Similar modification of the appearance of CMV pneumonitis is seen in patients partly treated at the time of biopsy. It is very unusual to see these changes whilst taking prophylaxis and patient compliance should be checked.

In some biopsies CMV pneumonitis is seen with the additional features of mononuclear infiltrates more typical of acute rejection. This may represent concomitant viral pneumonitis with rejection which precludes grading and the decision to treat either or both processes can be difficult. These patients often require follow-up biopsy to confirm appropriate treatment and response. Prophylaxis has 'postponed' CMV pneumonitis to an intermediate or late graft complication rather than early. Concomitant acute rejection which is a feature of the early postoperative period is therefore seen less frequently. The effect of this postponement on survival and development of obliterative bronchiolitis has yet to be evaluated.

Table 7

Features of acute rejection and CMV pneumonitis

Acute rejection	CMV pneumonitis
Tight perivascular infiltrates, mainly mononuclear cells	Infiltrates not tightly perivascular; usually in external adventitia only
Polymorphs and eosinophils in moderate – severe grade	Polymorphs common and may predominate; eosinophils rare; polymorphs in alveolar walls
Perivascular edema absent or mild	Perivascular edema prominent
No microabscesses	Microabscesses common
Alveolar cell hyperplasia in high-grade rejection	Alveolar cell hyperplasia common
No viral inclusions	Intranuclear and intracytoplasmic viral inclusions in macrophages, alveolar and endothelial cells
Lymphocytic endothelialitis	Lymphocytes and polymorphs in endothelium, related to viral inclusions, but rare in biopsy material

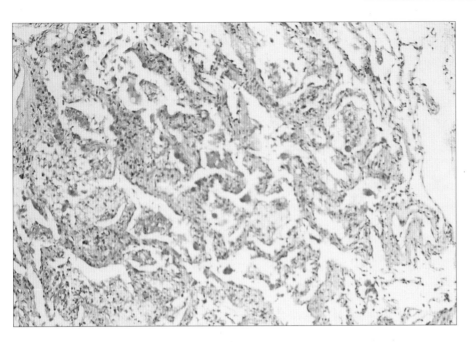

Figure 24.1
A low-power view of a transbronchial biopsy showing diffuse alveolitis with interstitial and intra-alveolar inflammation and abundant fibrin. In this florid case at low-power it is possible to identify enlarged alveolar epithelial cells and macrophages containing typical intranuclear inclusions of CMV. Nowhere in the biopsy is there evidence of a perivascular predilection for the inflammation.

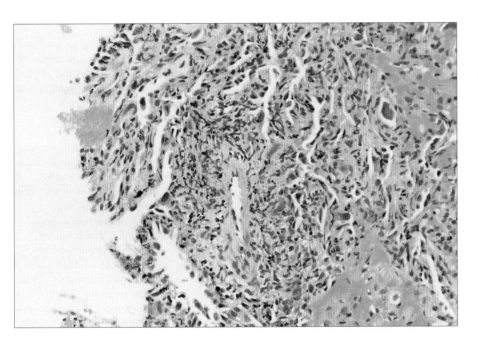

Figure 24.2
Transbronchial biopsy showing severe viral pneumonitis with diffuse infiltration including numerous polymorphs. There is fibrin and inflammatory cell infiltration of alveolar spaces. Easily visible at this power are the enlarged alveolar epithelial cells with hematoxyphilic intranuclear inclusions. The nature of the infiltrate with numerous polymorphs and its diffuse nature are quite unlike the infiltrates of acute lung rejection. This florid appearance of CMV pneumonitis is far less common since the introduction of ganciclovir prophylaxis.

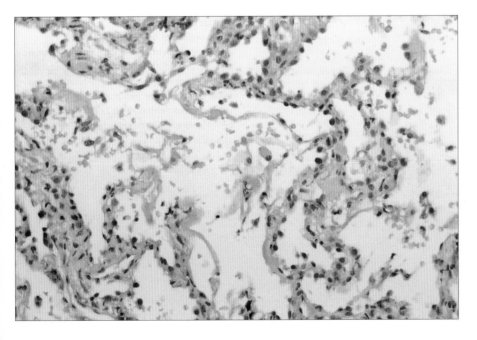

Figure 24.3
Transbronchial biopsy from a patient with CMV pneumonitis showing early hyaline membrane formation. This is an unusual feature in biopsy pathology as patients tend to present early in the natural history of the disease. Typical CMV inclusions were present in other fields. The patient was a CMV mismatch early in the transplant program, i.e. the seronegative recipient was given seropositive donor heart and lungs.

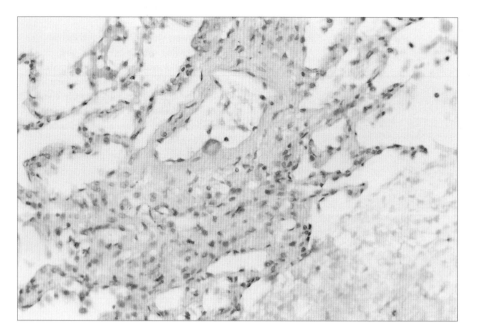

Figure 24.4

A transbronchial biopsy showing a CMV inclusion in an endothelial cell in a patient with typical CMV pneumonitis in other biopsy fragments. There is interstitial inflammation in this biopsy with polymorphs and mononuclear cells. Endothelial cell infection by CMV can induce an endothelialitis and cause diagnostic confusion with acute rejection. Attention to other features in the biopsy should however allow the correct diagnosis to be made. This is another instance where further serial sections into the biopsy may be necessary to investigate the abnormality.

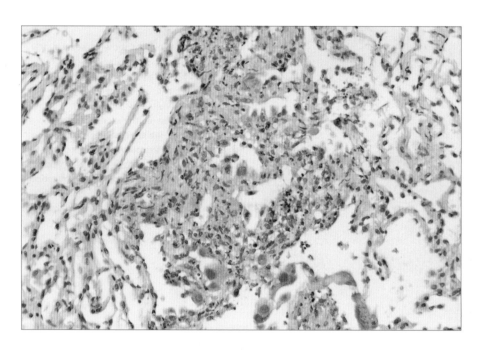

Figure 24.5

Transbronchial biopsy showing an alveolitis which involves parenchyma in the center of the field with relative sparing at the margins. The predominant inflammatory cell is the neutrophil with microabscess formation. Numerous enlarged alveolar epithelial cells with intranuclear hemotoxyphilic inclusions characteristic of CMV are readily identified. This appearance contrasts with the diffuse viral alveolitis seen prior to prophylaxis and is much more of a focal neutrophilic alveolitis. It is therefore critical for the correct diagnosis of opportunistic infection that adequate parenchymal samples are submitted for microscopy. In the absence of diagnostic inclusions focal neutrophilic alveolitis should raise a high index of suspicion of CMV pneumonitis. Serology and CMV antigenemia may be helpful in diagnosis.

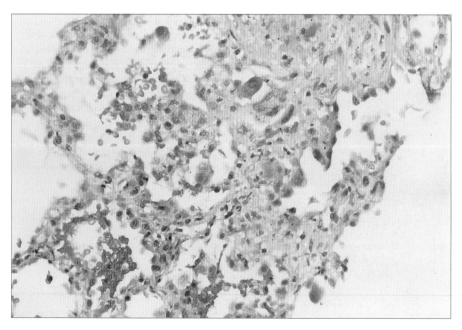

Figure 24.6

Transbronchial biopsy showing CMV pneumonitis with diagnostic viral inclusions in a setting of alveolitis with inflammatory cells, hemorrhage and type II pneumocyte hyperplasia. Cases like this do not require immunocytochemistry for confirmation being entirely diagnostic on biopsy appearance.

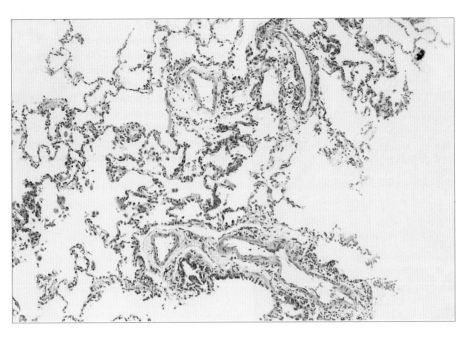

Figure 24.7
Transbronchial biopsy from a patient with CMV alveolitis. This low-power view shows some thickening of the alveolar walls focally which contained polymorphs. The vessels at this power show prominent perivascular edema with no evidence of inflammatory cell cuffing. This edema is a consistent feature of CMV pneumonitis and the appearance of the vessels is helpful in distinguishing infiltrates from those of acute rejection.

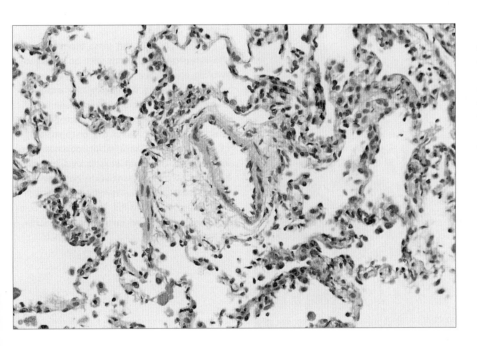

Figure 24.8
A higher power view of the same biopsy shows the lack of perivascular cuffing by inflammatory cells and emphasizes the edema. The adjacent alveolar walls show thickening with neutrophils infiltrating and type II pneumocytes being prominent. No diagnostic CMV inclusions are present in this field. They were numerous in other parts of the biopsy.

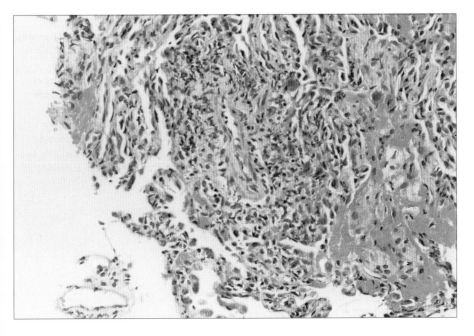

Figure 24.9
Active CMV alveolitis in this transbronchial biopsy is associated with some lymphocytes attached to the endothelium of the central vessel. Serial sections failed to reveal viral infection of endothelial cells. The most likely cause is the CMV pneumonitis, but acute rejection enters the differential diagnosis. No other perivascular distribution of infiltrates was seen in the serially sectioned fragments and the patient made a full recovery on antiviral therapy.

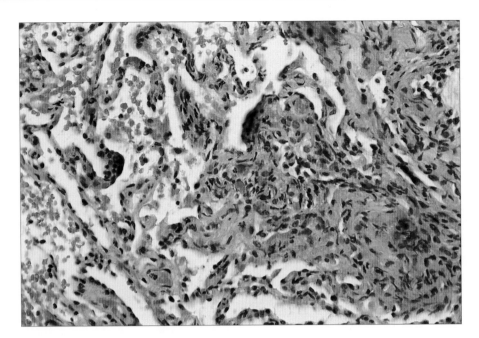

Figure 24.10
Transbronchial biopsy from a patient suspected of developing CMV following cessation of prophylaxis. The parenchyma is diffusely abnormal with inflammatory infiltrate showing polymorphs. There is type II cell hyperplasia and a single enlarged alveolar epithelial cell in the center of the field with an intranuclear inclusion within an area of polymorph infiltration consistent with CMV.

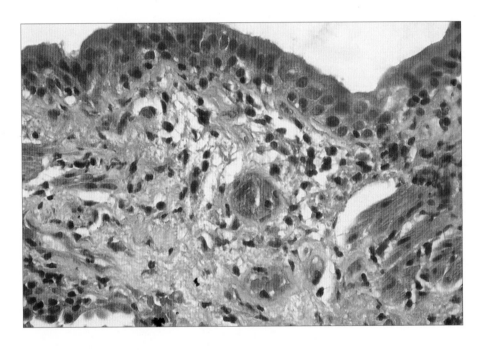

Figure 24.11
A mucosal piece in the same biopsy series shows normal epithelium with an enlarged swollen endothelial cell in an airway vessel with a degenerate hematoxyphilic inclusion and cytoplasmic granularity consistent with CMV. This degenerate appearance of the infected cell is typical of the histopathology of CMV following antiviral prophylaxis. The involvement of airway vessels by CMV may be relevant to the association between CMV disease and the development of obliterative bronchiolitis. We have not seen bronchiolar epithelial involvement by CMV in lung allografts.

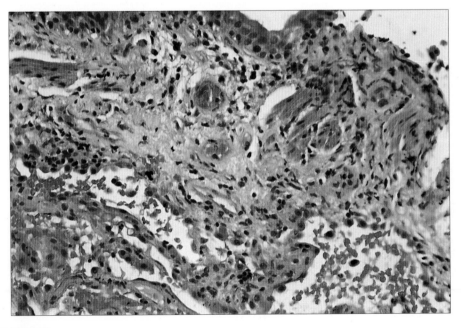

Figure 24.12
A lower power view shows the relationship of this abnormal vessel to the peribronchiolar parenchyma which is severely inflamed. The relative sparing of the airway itself is characteristic of CMV pneumonitis and a helpful differential diagnostic feature from herpes simplex infection of the graft. It is uncommon to identify CMV in airway vessels like this and the importance of high-power screening of all biopsy material cannot be overemphasized.

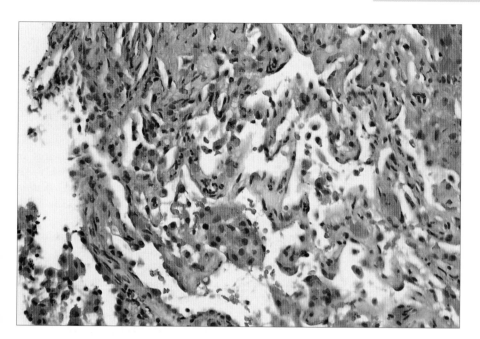

Figure 24.13
The parenchymal changes in this case of CMV pneumonitis following prophylaxis appear rather non-specific. The neutrophilic infiltration of alveolar walls is however much more characteristic of infection than rejection.

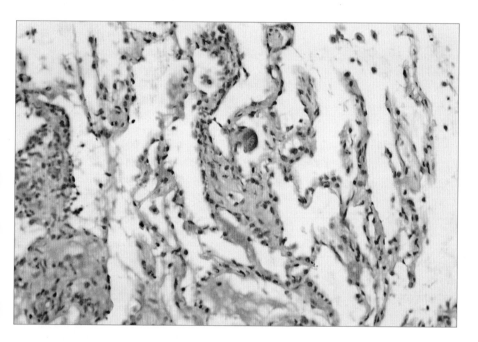

Figure 24.14
Focal neutrophilic alveolitis involving alveolar walls with minor changes only in alveolar spaces. An alveolar epithelial cell contains a degenerate intranuclear inclusion of cytomegalovirus. Cytoplasmic inclusions can also be discerned. This episode of CMV pneumonitis occurred following a period of prophylaxis and is now the commonest form of CMV pneumonitis in our experience. It is not always visible at scanning magnification. Each biopsy fragment must therefore be carefully screened.

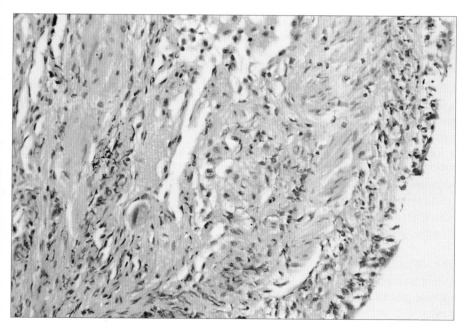

Figure 24.15
A degenerate CMV intranuclear inclusion is present in an enlarged cell probably of endothelial origin in an airway which shows acute inflammation of the epithelial surface. There is no evidence of CMV inclusions elsewhere but serologic changes and polymerase chain reaction indicated active CMV infection for which treatment was given. The bronchial epithelial changes are related to concomitant bacterial airways infection rather than a direct CMV effect. Superimposed bacterial infections are common in CMV pneumonitis.

FURTHER READING

Arbustini E, Morbini P, Grasso M *et al.* Human cytomegalovirus early infection, acute rejection, and major histocompatibility class II antigen expression in the transplanted lung. *Transplantation* 1996; **61**:418–27.

Bailey TC, Trulock EP, Ettinger NA, Storch GA, Cooper JD, Powderly WG. Failure of prophylactic gancyclovir to prevent cytomegalovirus disease in recipients of lung transplants. *J Infect Dis* 1992;**165**:548–52.

Beck S, Barrell BG. Human cytomegalovirus encodes a glycoprotein homologous to MHC class-I antigens. *Nature* 1998;**331**:269–72.

Burke CM, Glanville AR, Macoviak JA. The spectrum of cytomegalovirus infection in human heart-lung transplantation. *J Heart Transplant* 1986;**5**:267–72.

Cooper J D, Billingham M, Egan T *et al.* A working formulation for the standardization of nomenclature and for clinical staging of chronic dysfunction in lung allografts. *J Heart Lung Transplant* 1993;**12**:713–16.

Craigen JL, Grundy JE. Cytomegalovirus induced up-regulation of LFA-3 (CD58) and ICAM-1 (CD54) is a direct viral effect that is not prevented by Ganciclovir or Foscarnet treatment. *Transplantation* 1996;**62**:1102–8.

Duncan AJ, Dummer JS, Paradis IL *et al.* Cytomegalovirus infection and survival in lung transplant recipients. *J Heart Lung Transplant* 1991;**10**:638–46.

Duncan SR, Paradis IL, Yousem SA *et al.* Sequelae of cytomegalovirus pulmonary infections in lung allograft recipients. *Am Rev Respir Dis* 1992;**146**:1419–25.

Egan JJ, Barber L, Lomax J *et al.* Detection of human cytomegalovirus antigenaemia: a rapid diagnostic technique for predicting cytomegalovirus infection/pneumonitis in lung and heart transplant recipients. *Thorax* 1995;**50**:9–13.

Ettinger NA, Bailey TC, Trulock EP *et al.* Cytomegalovirus Infection and Pneumonitis: Impact After Isolated Lung Transplantation. *Am Rev Respir Dis* 1993;**147**:1017–23.

Flint A, Frank TS. Cytomegalovirus detection in lung transplant biopsy samples by polymerase chain reaction. *J Heart Lung Transplant* 1994;**13**:38–42.

Gerbase MW, Dubois D, Rothmeier C, Spiliopoulos A, Wunderli W, Nicod LP. Costs and outcomes of prolonged cytomegalovirus prophylaxis to cover the enhanced immunosuppression phase following lung transplantation. *Chest* 1999;**116**:1265–72.

Gould FK, Freeman R, Taylor CE, Ashcroft T, Dark JH, Corris PA. Prophylaxis and management of cytomegalovirus pneumonitis after lung transplantation: a review of experience in one centre. *J Heart Lung Transplant* 1993;**12**:695–9.

Gutiérrez CA, Chaparro C, Krajden M, Winton T, Kesten S. Cytomegalovirus viremia in lung transplant recipients receiving ganciclovir and immune globulin. *Chest* 1998;**113**:924–32.

Ho M. Observations from transplantation contributing to the understanding of pathogenesis of CMV infection. *Transplant Proc* 1991;**23**:104–9.

Humbert M, Devergne O, Cerrina J *et al.* Activation of macrophages and cytotoxic cells during cytomegalovirus pneumonia complicating lung transplants. *Am Rev Respir Dis* 1992;**145**:1178–184.

Hutter JA, Scott JP, Wreghitt T, Higenbottam T, Wallwork J. The importance of cytomegalovirus in heart-lung transplant recipients. *Chest* 1989;**95**:627–31.

Katzenstein AL, Askin FB. *Surgical pathology of non-neoplastic lung disease.* 1990; pp. 326–333. W B Saunders, Philadelphia.

Keenan RJ, Lega ME, Dummer S *et al.* Cytomegalovirus serologic status and postoperative infection correlated with risk of developing chronic rejection after pulmonary transplantation. *Transplantation* 1991;**51**:433–8.

Koskinen PK, Kallio EA, Bruggeman CA, Lembström K. Cytomegalovirus infection enhances experimental obliterative bronchiolitis in rat tracheal allograft. *Am J Respir Crit Care Med* 1997;**155**:2078–88.

Myerson D, Hackman RC, Nelson JA, Ward DC, McDougall JK. Widespread presence of histologically occult cytomegalovirus. *Hum Pathol* 1984;**15**:430–39.

Nakhleh RE, Bolman RM, Henke CA, Hertz MI. Lung transplant pathology. A comparative study of pulmonary acute rejection and cytomegalovirus infection. *Am J Surg Pathol* 1991;**15**:1197–1201.

Niedobitek G, Finn T, Herbst H *et al.* Detection of cytomegalovirus by *in-situ* hybridisation and histochemistry using a monoclonal antibody CCH2: a comparison of methods. *J Clin Path* 1988; **41**:1005–1009.

Orens JB. Cytomegalovirus prophylaxis with IV ganciclovir in lung transplant recipients. The long and the short of it. *Chest* 1999;**116**:1153–3.

Revello MG, Percivalle E, Arbustini E, Pardi R, Sozzani S, Gerna G. *In vitro* generation of human cytomegalovirus pp65 antigenaemia, viremia, and leukoDNAemia. *J Clin Invest* 1998;**101**:2686–92.

Smyth RL, Scott JP, Borysiewicz LK *et al.* Cytomegalovirus infection in heart–lung transplant recipients: risk factors, clinical associations and response to treatment. *J Infect Dis* 1991; **164**:1045–50.

Smyth RL, Sinclair J, Scott JP *et al.* Infection and reactivation with cytomegalovirus strains in lung transplant recipients. *Transplantation* 1991;**52**:480–1.

Soghikian MV, Valentine VG, Berry GJ, Patel HR, Robbins RC, Theodore J. Impact of gancyclovir prophylaxis on heart–lung and lung transplant recipients. *J Heart Lung Transplant* 1996;**15**:881–7.

Strickler JG, Manivel C, Copenhaver CM, Kubic VL. Comparison of *in situ* hybridisation and immunohistochemistry for detection of cytomegalovirus and herpes simplex virus. *Hum Pathol* 1990;**21**:443–8.

Theise ND, Haber MM, Grimes MM. Detection of cytomegalovirus in lung allografts. Comparison of histologic and immunohistochemical findings. *Am J Clin Pathol* 1991;**96**:762–6.

von Willebrand E, Pettersson E, Ahonen J, Hayry P. Cytomegalovirus infection, class II expression and rejection during the course of cytomegalovirus disease. *Transplant Proc* 1986;**18**:32–4.

Weiss LM, Movahed LA, Berry GJ, Billingham ME. *In situ* hybridization studies for viral nucleic acids in heart and lung allograft biopsies. *Am J Clin Pathol* 1990;**93**:675–79.

Wreghitt TG, Hakim M, Gray JJ, Kucia S, Wallwork J. Cytomegalovirus infections in heart and heart and lung transplant recipients. *J Clin Pathol* 1988;**41**:660–67.

Wreghitt TG, Smyth RL, Scott JP *et al*. Value of culture of biopsy material in diagnosis of viral infections in heart–lung transplant recipients. *Transplant Proc* 1990;**22**:1809–1810.

HERPES SIMPLEX PNEUMONITIS

Herpes simplex infection in lung transplant patients generally follows a period of augmented immunosuppression and with effective prophylactic regimes is very uncommon in current practice. It is a bronchopneumonic process with distribution around airways and adjoining air spaces. The inflammation includes numerous polymorphs with abundant pyknosis and debris together with bronchial and bronchiolar epithelial necrosis. There may be hyaline membrane formation and interstitial edema and hemorrhage. The diagnostic inclusions are not easily found in biopsy material unless the samples have a good yield of small airways. The accompanying lavage however is often more informative with typical intranuclear inclusions in the shed epithelial cells accompanied by much pyknotic debris. Ground glass change and multinucleation is not frequent in herpes simplex virus (HSV) infection of the respiratory tract and in the presence of degenerative changes immunohistochemical methods may be useful. Herpes simplex virus infection does not produce cytoplasmic inclusions which together with lack of cell

enlargement are useful discriminators from CMV (Table 8). Occasionally both viral infections will co-exist and identification requires immunohistochemical or *in situ* methods for a definite diagnosis.

Herpes simplex virus infection is usually limited to patients who are seropositive prior to transplantation. This implies that the immunosuppressive regimes promote reactivation of latent viral infection rather than reinfection. Information about mucocutaneous lesions of herpes simplex including pharyngeal and tracheobronchial involvement is very helpful for the reporting pathologist. Routine samples of bronchoalveolar lavage fluid should always be sent for virologic assessment including immunofluorescent assay for confirmation of cytologic and histologic findings. Unfortunately HSV may be fatal with disseminated unsuspected disease discovered at autopsy. A high index of suspicion should be maintained particularly in the presence of hemorrhagic inflammation of the respiratory tract at bronchoscopy.

Table 8
Histologic features of CMV and HSV infection

	CMV	HSV
Viral inclusions	Intranuclear*	Intranuclear
	Hematoxyphilic	Eosinophilic
	'Owl's eye'	Dense nuclear membrane
	Halo	May be multiple
	Single	Multinucleation unusual
	Intracytoplasmic	No cytoplasmic inclusions
	Eosinophilic	
	Granular	
Infected cells	Alveolar epithelial	Bronchial epithelial
	Endothelial	Metaplastic squames
	Alveolar macrophages	Alveolar epithelial (rare)
Distribution	Interstitial pneumonitis	Bronchopneumonic pattern
	DAD	DAD
Inflammatory cells	Mononuclear with prominent polymorphs	Polymorphs with suppuration
	Microabsesses	Microabscesses
	Necrosis uncommon	Abundant necrosis with pyknosis

*Less pronounced after prophylaxis. DAD: Diffuse alveolar damage.

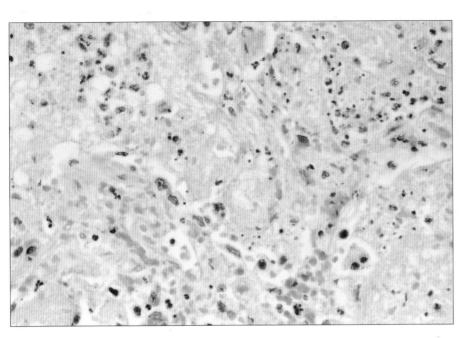

Figure 25.1
Autopsy lung with herpes simplex pneumonia which presented with new lung nodules and fever. The intense necrosis with intranuclear viral inclusions is typical and the diagnosis was confirmed by culture. HSV hepatitis was also present.

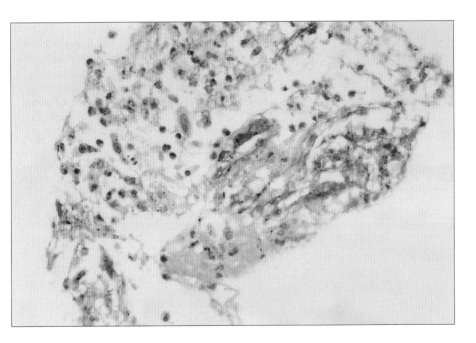

Figure 25.2
Mucosal debris with inflammatory cells in a patient with mucocutaneous herpes simplex lesions. The tracheobronchial tree was reddened at bronchoscopy and degenerate intraepithelial inclusions can be seen. These are consistent with HSV which was cultured from lavage and biopsy tissue.

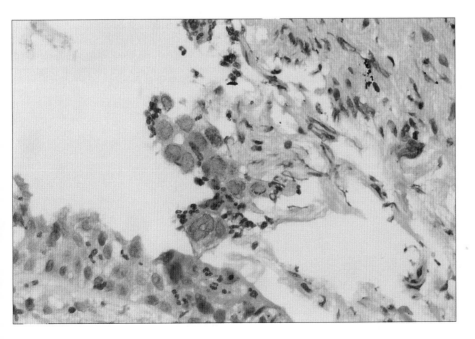

Figure 25.3
Intact bronchial epithelium showing typical ground-glass intranuclear inclusions of HSV. No cytoplasmic inclusions are present and there is no cellular enlargement.
Polymorphs are present in the virus-infected epithelium.

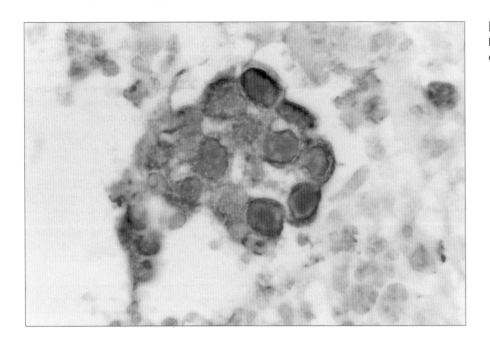

Figure 25.4
Immunoperoxidase staining for HSV confirms the diagnosis of Fig. 25.3.

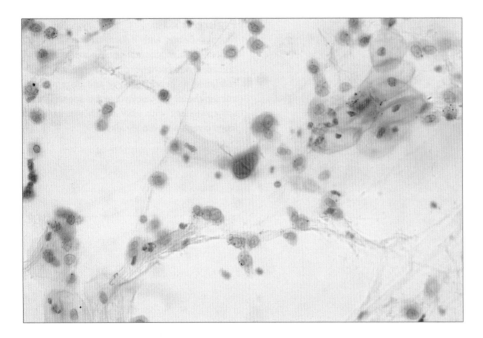

Figure 25.5
Lavage fluid stained by H & E shows herpes simplex ground-glass intranuclear inclusions with a halo. No mucocutaneous or pharyngeal lesions were present. The patient's respiratory symptoms responded to acyclovir, having followed a period of augmented immunosuppression.

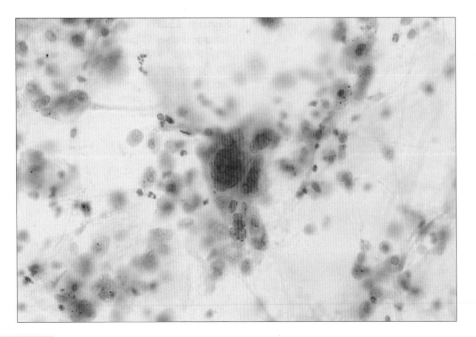

Figure 25.6
This case (same as Fig. 25.5) unusually shows frequent multinucleate virally-infected epithelial cells which are helpful in diagnosis. This pattern is not often seen in the respiratory tract.

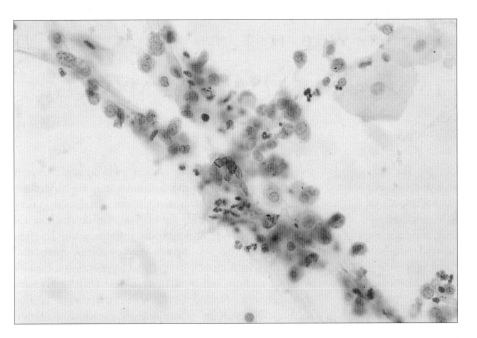

Figure 25.7
Lavage cytology demonstrates viral inclusions of HSV in the center of the field. The inclusions are pale, eosinophilic, ground-glass in type with a halo and dense nuclear membrane. The absence of cytomegaly requires diligent screening to make the diagnosis. The positive cytology may be the first indication of HSV.

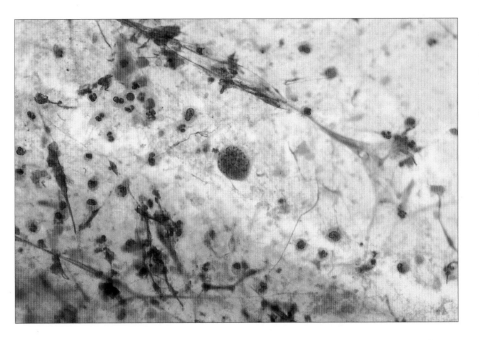

Figure 25.8
The bronchial aspirate in HSV infection is extremely necrotic with numerous polymorphs and debris. The causative organism may be overlooked especially if the virally-infected cells are degenerate as shown here. Intensely necrotic aspirates may require microbiological correlation as the yield of HSV in transbronchial biopsies is very low. Macrophage with pytnotic debris in center of field.

FURTHER READING

Byers RJ, Hasleton PS, Quigley A *et al*. Pulmonary herpes simplex in burns patients. *Eur Respir J* 1996;8:2313–17.

Geradts J, Warnock M, Yen B. Use of the polymerase chain reaction in the diagnosis of unsuspected herpes simplex viral pneumonia: Report of a case. *Hum Pathol* 1990;**21**:118–21.

Saral R, Burns WH, Laskin OL, Santos GW, Lietman PS. Acyclovir prophylaxis of herpes simplex virus infections. *N Engl J Med* 1981;305:3–67.

Smyth RL, Higenbottam TW, Scott JP *et al*. Herpes simplex virus infection in heart–lung transplant recipients. *Transplantation* 1990;**49**:735–39.

Weiss LM, Movahed LA, Berry GJ, Billingham ME. *In situ* hybridization studies for viral nucleic acids in heart and lung allograft biopsies. *Am J Clin Pathol* 1990;**93**:675–79.

Pneumocystis carinii pneumonia (PCP) is far less common since the introduction of effective prophylaxis, but is still seen from time to time in patients unable to take the prophylactic agents or through non-compliance. Lung allograft recipients commonly produce an atypical histologic reaction to PCP compared with the characteristic abundant intra-alveolar foamy exudate seen in other immunosuppressed patients in which cysts and trophozooites can be readily found. The transplanted lung usually shows granulomatous PCP with a paucity of organisms. In this setting, PCP is easily overlooked and should be sought with diligence in post transplant biopsies showing granulomatous inflammation. Silver staining of more than one serial section may be required together with immunohistochemical techniques. The granulomatous inflammation is often accompanied by an intense mononuclear interstitial infiltrate which closely mimics acute rejection although without endothelialitis in most cases. Diffuse alveolar damage as a reaction to *Pneumocystis carinii* is also seen rarely in lung transplant recipients and should prompt a diligent search for diagnostic cysts.

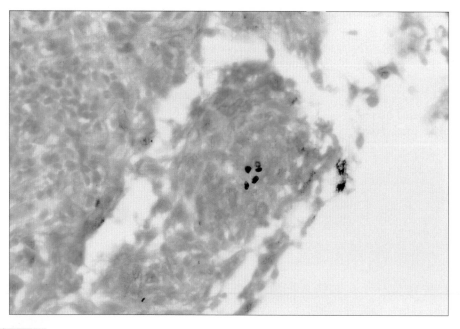

Figure 26.1
Transbronchial biopsy showing bronchiolar mucosal surface and numerous confluent non-caseating epithelioid cell and giant cell granulomas in peribronchiolar parenchyma. There is no evidence of foamy or honeycomb exudate within the granulomas. Grocott silver staining revealed pneumocysts.

Figure 26.2
Grocott silver stained section showing cluster of typical pneumocysts within a granuloma. Not all granulomas in the biopsy showed organisms. Granulomatous *Pneumocystis carinii* is the commonest form of *Pneumocystis* pneumonia in lung transplant recipients.

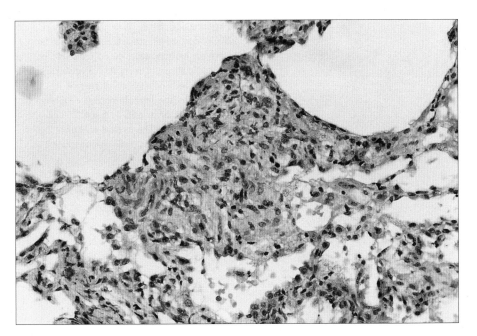

Figure 26.3
Transbronchial biopsy showing loosely formed granuloma with epithelioid cells but no giant cells deep within the parenchyma and associated with a non-specific inflammatory cell infiltration of alveolar walls. Occasional polymorphs and eosinophils are seen in this interstitial infiltrate. The granulomas were caused by *Pneumocystis carinii* pneumonia.

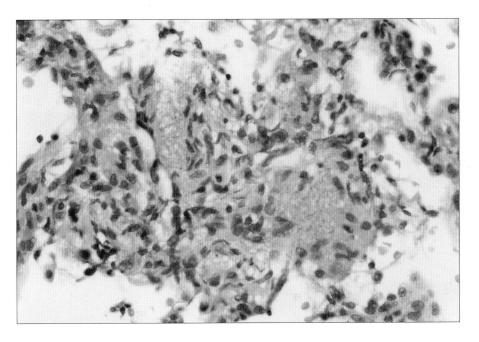

Figure 26.4
Another case of granulomatous *Pneumocystis* in a lung transplant recipient in which a single field shows typical foamy honeycomb exudate associated with the epithelioid cells of a loosely formed granuloma. This exudate revealed pneumocysts on silver staining.

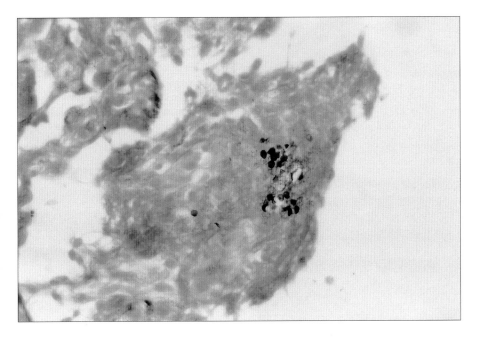

Figure 26.5
Grocott silver stain shows abundant pneumocysts in the exudate seen in Fig. 26.4. This number of easily found pneumocysts is rather unusual in lung transplantation pathology, where there is typically a florid inflammatory response to few organisms with an allografted organ.

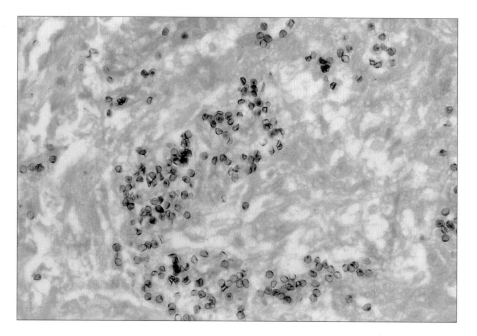

Figure 26.6
A Grocott silver stain transbronchial biopsy from an immunosuppressed leukemic patient for comparison. The typical alveolar exudate teeming with pneumocysts seen is in contrast to the granulomatous response to a paucity of organisms in lung transplantation. The typical morphology of the pneumocysts is well-demonstrated in this case.

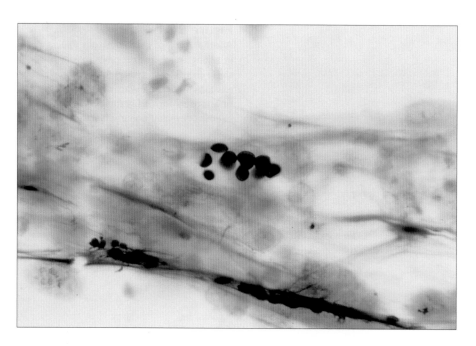

Figure 26.7
The accompanying bronchial lavage may demonstrate scanty pneumocysts as shown here in a lung transplant recipient. The cysts are round, oval and collapsed with helmet shaped forms also. Silver staining of the lavage is a rapid method of identifying the pneumocysts.

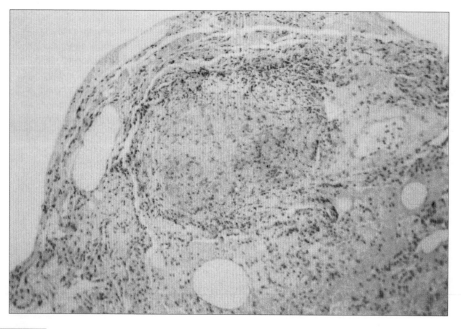

Figure 26.8
Transbronchial biopsy showing a large non-caseating epithelioid and giant cell granuloma in a transbronchial biopsy. No infectious agent was present either histologically, microbiologically or cytologically at this time and the cause of the granulomatous inflammation was unascertained.

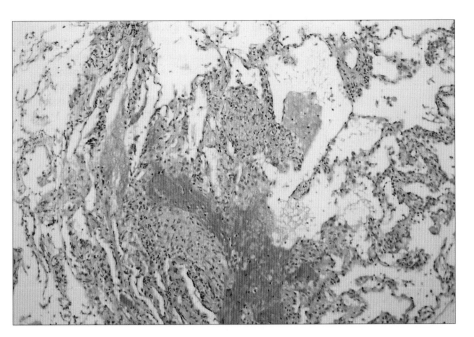

Figure 26.9
Transbronchial biopsy from the same patient 8 weeks later showing granulomatous inflammation with some fibrin and hemorrhage. The granulomas occupy a perivascular position on this occasion.

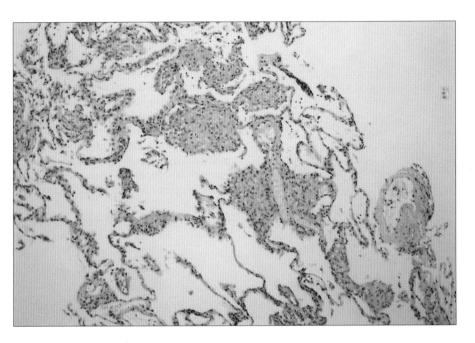

Figure 26.10
Low-power of the same transbronchial biopsy shows that the granulomas are perivascular in distribution and should not be confused with the infiltrates of acute rejection. Intra-alveolar granulomas are also present.

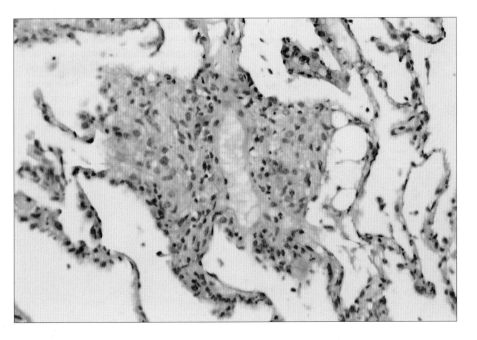

Figure 26.11
High-power view of same biopsy showing loosely formed granulomas around a thin-walled vessel with mononuclear cells and occasional polymorphs. Lymphocytes on the endothelium raise the possibility of endothelialitis but there are no other features to indicate acute rejection.

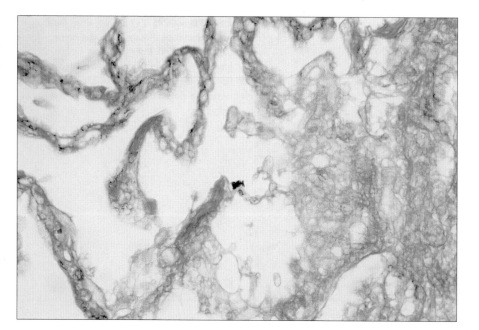

Figure 26.12
Grocott silver stain of same biopsy showing scanty pneumocysts in the center of the field. This is a case of granulomatous *Pneumocystis* pneumonia. The granulomas in Fig. 26.8 where *Pneumocystis* was not identified remain unexplained, but are likely to have been due to *Pneumocystis* which was not detected by any technique.

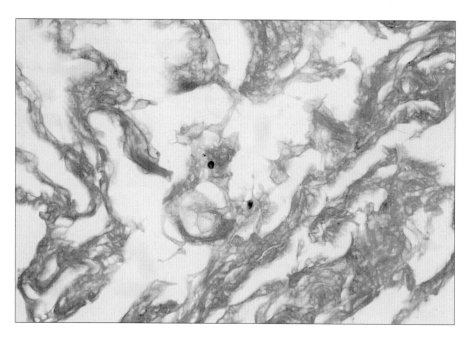

Figure 26.13
A single pneumocyst was present in this biopsy fragment with granulomatous inflammation. The typical morphology allows confident diagnosis, but high-power screening is essential in order not to miss the scanty organisms. The role of immunohistochemical and molecular techniques in the setting of such scanty pneumocysts is not fully evaluated. Silver staining with diligent screening will yield an earlier diagnosis in most cases.

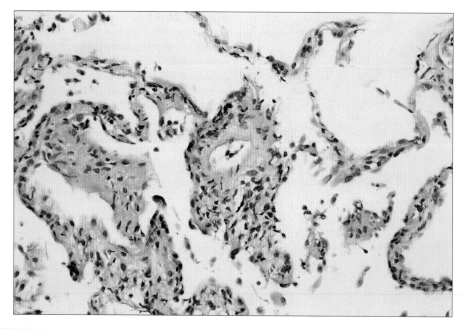

Figure 26.14
Elsewhere in the same transbronchial biopsy the granulomatous component is less prominent and the infiltrates can be easily confused with acute rejection. *Pneumocystis carinii* pneumonia is a very important mimic of acute rejection and should always be considered in the differential diagnosis.

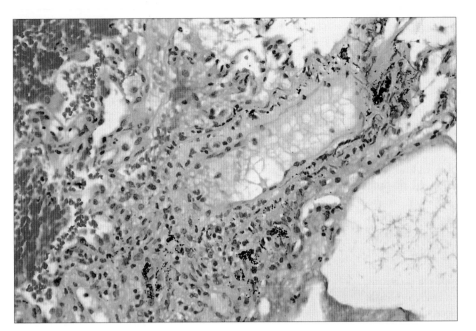

Figure 26.15
Another vessel in the biopsy showing granulomatous *Pneumocystis* pneumonia. This vessel shows a definite endothelialitis and there are occasional eosinophils in the infiltrate. This was considered to be part of the inflammatory response to *Pneumocystis* and was not treated with augmented immunosuppression. The patient responded fully to antimicrobial therapy, although histologically concomitant acute rejection cannot be absolutely excluded.

FURTHER READING

Blumenfeld W, McCook O, Holodniy M, Katzenstein DA. Correlation of morphologic diagnosis of *Pneumocystis carinii* with the presence of pneumocystis DNA amplified by the polymerase chain reaction. *Mod Pathol* 1992;**5**:103–106.

Golden JA, Hollander H, Stulbarg MS, Gamsu G. Bronchoalveolar lavage as the exclusive diagnostic modality for *Pneumocystis carinii* pneumonia. *Chest* 1986;**90**:18–22.

Gryzan S, Paradis IL, Zeevi A *et al.* Unexpectedly high incidence of *Pneumocystis carinii* infection after heart-lung transplantation: implications for lung defence and allograft survival. *Am Rev Resp Dis* 1988;**137**:1268–74.

Kramer MR, Stoehr C, Lewiston NJ, Starnes VA, Theodore J. Trimethoprim-Sulfamethoxazole prophylaxis for *Pneumocystis carinii* infections in heart–lung transplantation – how effective and for how long? *Transplantation* 1992;**53**:586–9.

Ognibene FP, Shelhamer J, Gill V *et al.* The diagnosis of *Pneumocystis carinii* pneumonia in patients with the acquired immunodeficiency syndrome using subsegmental bronchoalveolar lavage. *Am Rev Respir Dis* 1984;**129**:929–32.

Travis WD, Pittaluga S, Lipschik GY *et al.* Atypical pathologic manifestations of *Pneumocystis carinii* pneumonia in the acquired immune deficiency syndrome. *Am J Surg Pathol* 1990;**14**:615–25.

Vestbo J, Nielsen TL, Junge J, Lundgren JD. Amount of *Pneumocystis carinii* and degree of acute lung inflammation in HIV-associated *P carinii* pneumonia. *Chest* 1993;**104**:109–13.

Wakefield AE, Miller RF, Guiver LA, Hopkin JM. Granulomatous *Pneumocystis carinii* pneumonia: DNA amplification studies on bronchoscopic alveolar lavage samples. *J Clin Pathol* 1994;**47**:664–6.

Weber WR, Askin FB, Dehner LP. Lung biopsy in *Pneumocystis carinii* pneumonia. A histological study of typical and atypical features. *Am J Clin Pathol* 1977;**67**:11–19.

MYCOBACTERIAL INFECTION

Mycobacterial infection with both tuberculous and non-tuberculous organisms is now well-recognized in lung transplant recipients. The incidence appears to be increasing mainly as a result of increased survival of patients and a broader range of primary conditions leading to transplantation. Typical granulomatous inflammation with or without necrosis is the usual transbronchial biopsy finding and multiple sections should be examined with Ziehl–Neelsen and modified Ziehl–Neelsen staining. Occasionally necrosis without granulomas is seen as in mycobacterial disease in non-immunocompromised patients and requires a high index of suspicion. We have seen this pattern with *Mycobacterium kansasii*. Pulmonary tuberculosis may be identified in the explanted lung(s) or native lung and may also be donor transmitted. Tuberculosis in the transplanted lung is still uncommon and has many pulmonary manifestations including nodules, bronchial narrowing, cavitation and pleural effusion. Atypical mycobacteria may colonize without disease and the role of therapy in simple colonization of the transplanted lung is unclear. Non-tuberculous mycobacterial infection may be an under-recognized cause of graft dysfunction. All forms of mycobacterial disease in the lung graft tend to be late and may occur in the setting of obliterative bronchiolitis. Mycobacterial infection is one of the *treatable* causes of symptoms for which transbronchial biopsies and lavage are performed in the context of known chronic rejection.

Patients whose primary diagnosis was sarcoidosis may undergo recurrence in the transplanted lung. Granulomas in transbronchial biopsy material even from these patients should be regarded as highly suspicious of opportunistic infection until proved otherwise. The need for parallel samples to be sent for microbiological assessment must be emphasized to the clinicians.

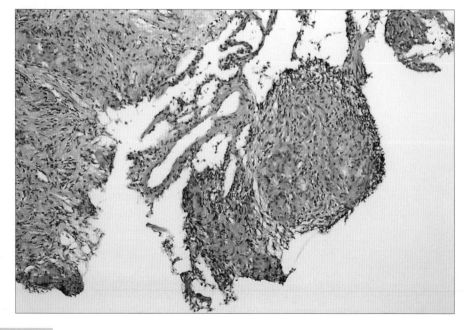

Figure 27.1
Transbronchial biopsy showing epithelioid granulomas without necrosis in a patient who developed *Mycobacterium tuberculosis* infection following lung transplantation. *Mycobacterium tuberculosis* was cultured from biopsy and lavage fluid.

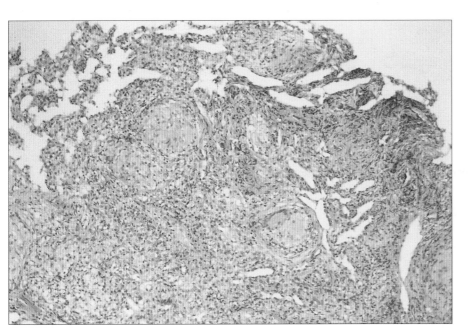

Figure 27.2
Transbronchial biopsy showing extensive granulomatous inflammation in interstitium with epithelioid cells and Langhans' giant cells. No evidence of necrosis is present. No organisms were demonstrated on Ziehl–Neelsen or modified Ziehl–Neelsen staining. *Mycobacterium kansasii* was later cultured from the aspirate, but not seen even retrospectively in the biopsy material.

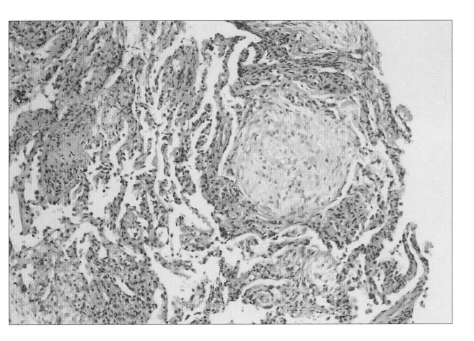

Figure 27.3
Transbronchial biopsy showing non-caseating epithelioid and giant cell granuloma distorting parenchyma. There is associated interstitial inflammation with mononuclear cells which are diffuse and not perivascular. Organisms were seen on special stains consistent with atypical mycobacteria. *Mycobacterium kansasii* was grown later from a biopsy fragment and lavage fluid.

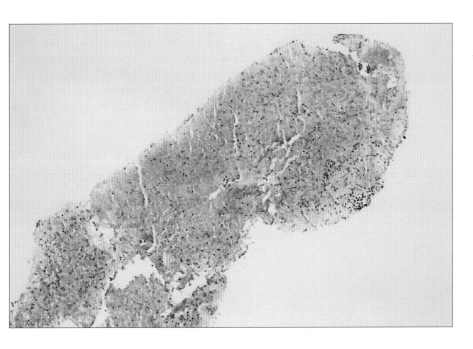

Figure 27.4
Needle core biopsy of lung nodule in transplanted lung showing necrosis but no granulomas. The patient had developed fever and a new peripheral lung nodule. (See Fig. 27.5.)

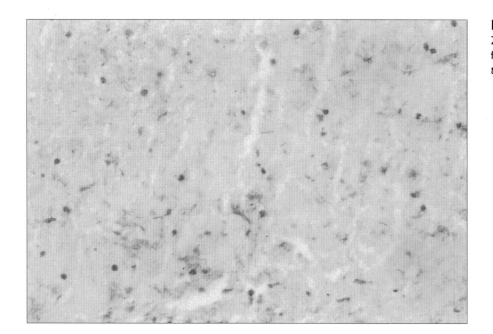

Figure 27.5
Ziehl–Neelsen staining shows numerous acid fast bacilli in this case of *Mycobacterium tuberculosis* which was confirmed on culture.

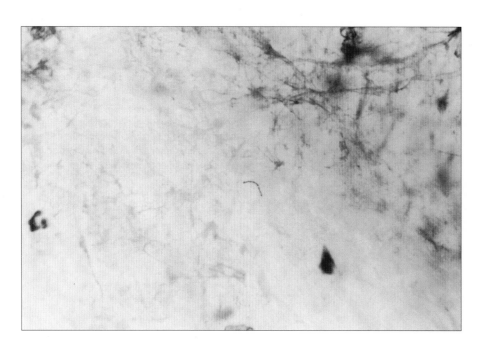

Figure 27.6
Ziehl–Neelsen staining of bronchial aspirate showing *Mycobacterium tuberculosis* which was also cultured.

FURTHER READING

Baldi S, Rapellino M, Ruffini E, Cavallo A, Mancuso M. Atypical mycobacteriosis in a lung transplant recipient. *Eur Respir J* 1997;**10**:952–4.

Baughman RP. Can tuberculosis cause sarcoidosis? *Chest* 1998;**114**:363–4.

Dromer C, Nashef SAM, Velly J-F, Martigne C, Couraud L. Tuberculosis in transplanted lungs. *J Heart Lung Transplant* 1993;**12**:924–7.

Kesten S, Chaparro C. Mycobacterial infections in lung transplant recipients. *Chest* 1999;**115**:741–5.

Malouf MA, Glanville AR. The spectrum of mycobacterial infection after lung transplantation. *Am J Respir Crit Care Med* 1999;**160**:1611–16.

Ridgeway AL, Warner G S, Phillips P *et al*. Transmission of *Mycobacterium tuberculosis* to recipients of single lung transplants from the same donor. *Am J Respir Crit Care Med* 1996;**153**:1166–8.

Schulman LL, Scully B, McGregor CC, Austin JHM. Pulmonary tuberculosis after lung transplantation. *Chest* 1997;**111**:1459–62.

Trulock EP, Bolman RM, Genton R. Pulmonary disease caused by mycobacterium chelonae in a heart–lung transplant recipient with obliterative bronchiolitis. *Am Rev Respir Dis* 1989;**140**:802–5.

Aspergillus has remained a major clinical problem in lung transplant programs over the years. This ubiquitous fungus causes a wide spectrum of disease ranging from simple colonization to invasive widely disseminated disease. Transbronchial biopsies and complementary lavage specimens should be interpreted together when *Aspergillus* infection is a possibility so that the correct diagnosis on the spectrum of disease can be made for the individual patients. Transbronchial biopsy appearances range from normal tissue to abundant eosinophil infiltration in those patients with allergic bronchopulmonary aspergillosis or may show mucoid impaction with eosinophilic pneumonia. Granulomas can be seen in the bronchocentric granulomatous mycosis with infrequent and fragmented fungal hyphae. Biopsies may also show cavitation with necrosis in invasive *Aspergillus* disease. The biopsies of bronchial and bronchiolar wall are often particularly informative in *Aspergillus* disease particularly in the early postoperative period when the relatively ischemic airway is prone to colonization and infection. Fragments of slough or degenerative cartilage should be carefully examined and stained on multiple sections in order to identify the *Aspergillus* hyphae and correlated with bronchoscopic appearances of the anastomosis. Fungal airway infections are far less common in combined heart–lung grafts with tracheal anastomoses which are well-vascularized (Table 9).

Fine needle aspiration biopsies of pulmonary nodules may be performed in patients with suspected *Aspergillus* infection and have a high diagnostic yield, particularly if CT guided.

Table 9

Patterns of *Aspergillus* infection in the transplanted lung

	Small airway	Parenchyma	Large airway
Non-invasive	Saprophytic colonization	Colonization of cavity	Saprophytic colonization Obstructive tracheobronchial aspergillosis
Minimally invasive	Bronchocentric granulomatous mycosis	Colonization of cavity; focal invasion of wall	Bronchocentric granulomatous mycosis
Invasive	*Aspergillus* bronchiolitis	Suppurative pneumonia with or without cavitation and abscess formation	Pseudomembranous tracheobronchitis Invasion of ischemic tracheobronchial wall *Aspergillus* bronchitis

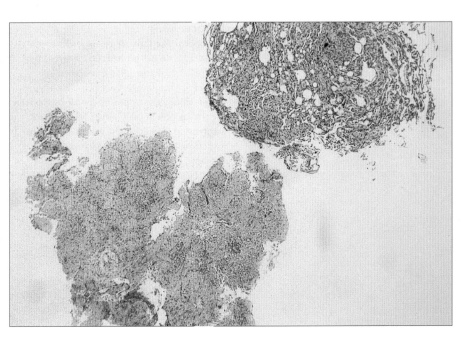

Figure 28.1

Transbronchial biopsies from a patient with a new cavitating lesion. One piece of lung parenchyma is viable with inflammatory cell infiltration. The other piece is clearly necrotic at low-power.

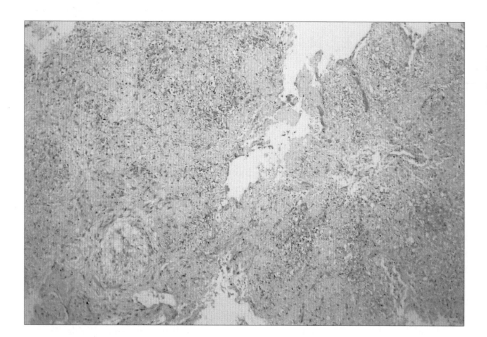

Figure 28.2
A higher power view of the necrotic area shows cellular debris with much pyknosis. The normal lung architecture is effaced but the cause of the necrosis is not clear at this magnification.

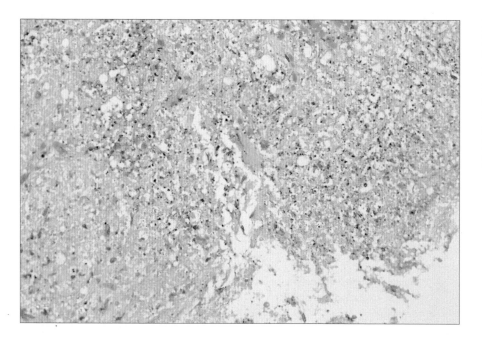

Figure 28.3
Higher power shows some faint haematoxyphilic hyphal structures which are consistent with *Aspergillus*, indicating that the cavity is due to *Aspergillus* pneumonia. Previous X-rays had been normal. It may not be possible in an individual patient to determine if the cavitation is due to the fungal infection or whether the cavity is pre-existing.

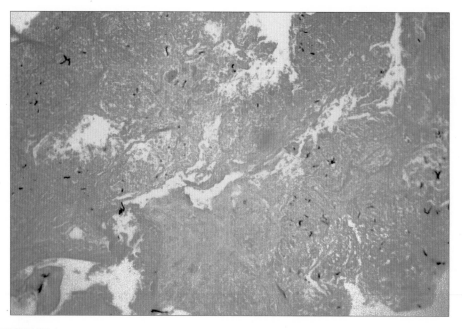

Figure 28.4
Grocott silver staining reveals numerous fungal hyphae in this necrotic fragment. *Aspergillus fumigatus* was confirmed on culture of the lavage fluid. This biopsy series shows the appearances of necrotizing *Aspergillus* pneumonia which followed augmented immunosuppression for acute rejection and responded to antifungal therapy.

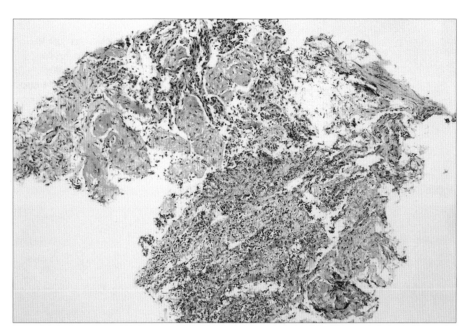

Figure 28.5
Transbronchial biopsy showing necrosis of lung parenchyma with fibrinous reaction in adjacent parenchyma. This biopsy also showed numerous *Aspergillus* hyphae, the pneumonia being due to invasive *Aspergillus*.

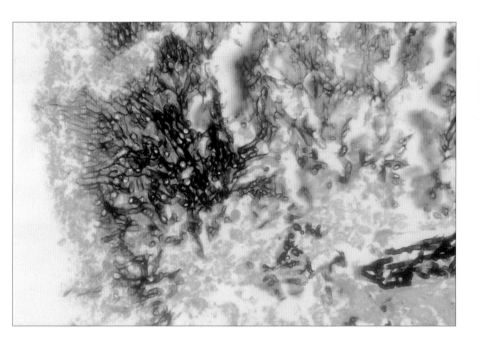

Figure 28.6
Grocott silver staining of Fig. 28.5 confirms large numbers of typical *Aspergillus* hyphae with dichotomous branching, transverse septa and regular hyphal thickness. These appearances are so characteristic that *Aspergillus* can be confidently diagnosed whilst awaiting culture.

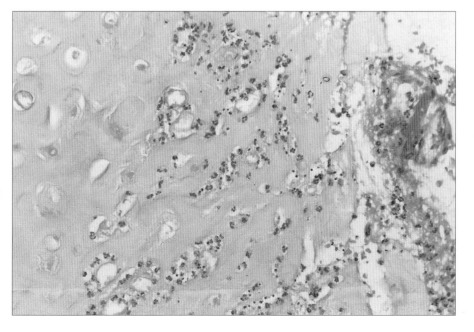

Figure 28.7
Ischemic cartilage with necrotic debris and polymorphs at its margin in a patient with an anastomotic problem postoperatively. Small numbers of fungal hyphae were present associated with inflammatory cells in the cartilage. The lavage contained abundant fungal hyphae. Fungus later eroded into pulmonary artery causing fatal hemorrhage. In other cases, antifungal therapy has prevented this complication. The best preventive strategy remains good surgical anastomotic technique with good vascularization of the airway.

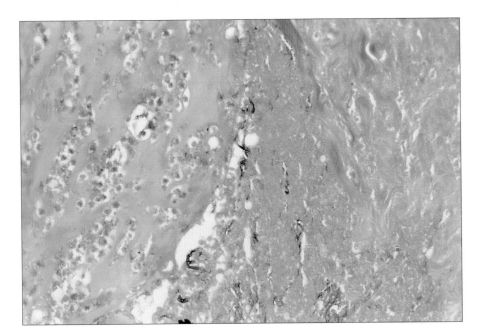

Figure 28.8
Grocott staining of necrotic cartilage to demonstrate frequent *Aspergillus* hyphae. The airway itself may dehisce, causing mediastinitis as well as risking erosion into major pulmonary vessels. Same case as Fig. 28.7.

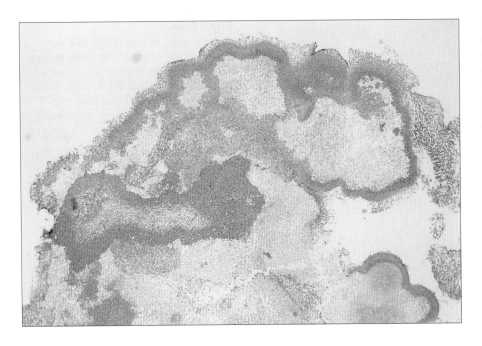

Figure 28.9
Section of tenacious material obstructing tracheobronchial tree and consisting entirely of *Aspergillus* hyphae. This is a condition called obstructing tracheobronchial aspergillosis (OBTA) which responded to bronchial toilet. There is no evidence of tissue invasion in this form of *Aspergillus* disease which is an extreme form of colonization.

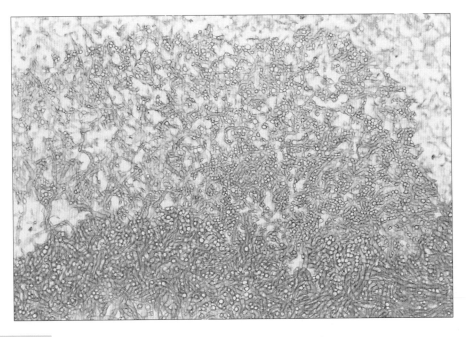

Figure 28.10
High-power of OBTA showing detailed morphology of the fungal hyphae which can be adequately assessed on H & E staining. Special fungal stains are required routinely in lung transplant biopsies to locate and identify the organisms. Tissue invasion cannot be reliably excluded by H & E alone.

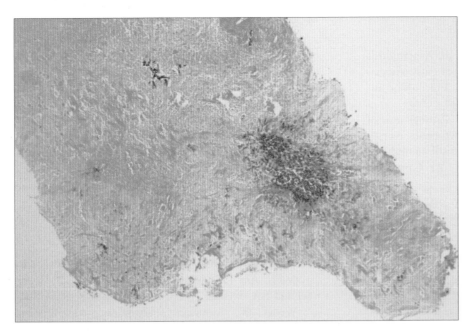

Figure 28.11
Needle core biopsy of new nodules in lung transplant showing *Aspergillus* on H & E staining. The nodules showed cavitation on CT which may be fungal in origin but small cavitating infarcts or even previous biopsy sites may become infected with *Aspergillus*. There was no previous radiologic evidence of parenchymal cavities however.

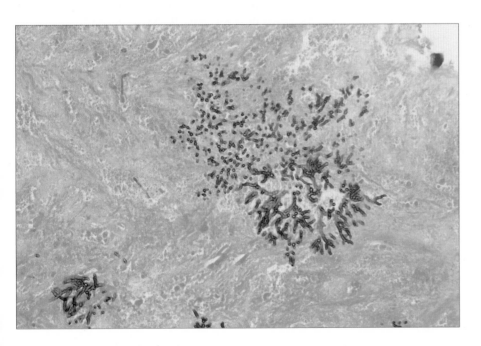

Figure 28.12
Grocott stain of needle core biopsy confirming the diagnosis. The nodules regressed on antifungal therapy in this case.

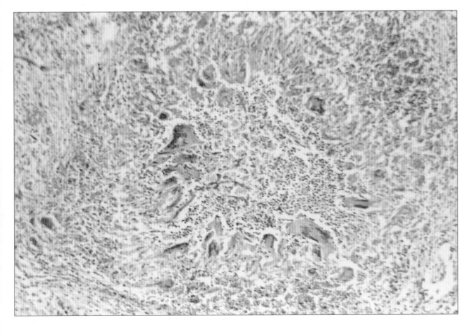

Figure 28.13
Bronchocentric granulomatous mycosis due to *Aspergillus* in a lung recipient. The bronchial wall is replaced by granulomatous tissue with obvious giant cells and the lumen contains inflammatory cells, mainly polymorphs. *Aspergillus* hyphae are also easily visible on the H & E stained section which is rather unusual. Often sparse, fragmented hyphae are only seen on special stains.

FURTHER READING

Anderson K, Morris G, Kennedy H *et al*. Aspergillosis in immunocompromised paediatric patients: associations with building hygiene, design, and indoor air. *Thorax* 1996;**51**:256–61.

Berenguer J, Allende MC, Lee JW *et al*. Pathogenesis of pulmonary aspergillosis. Granulocytopenia versus cyclosporine and methylprednisolone-induced immunosuppression. *Am J Respir Crit Care Med* 1995;**152**:1079–86.

Boon AP, O'Brien D, Adams DH. 10 year review of invasive aspergillosis detected at necropsy. *J Clin Pathol* 1991;**44**:452–4.

Cahill BC, Hibbs JR, Savik K *et al*. *Aspergillus* airway colonization and invasive disease after lung transplantation. *Chest* 1997;**112**:1160–64.

End A, Helbich T, Wisser W, Dekan G, Kleptoko W. The pulmonary nodule after lung transplantation. Cause and outcome. *Chest* 1995;**107**:1317–22.

Fitzsimons EJ, Aris R, Patterson R. Recurrence of allergic bronchopulmonary aspergillosis in the posttransplant lungs of a cystic fibrosis patient. *Chest* 1997;**112**: 281–2.

Hines DW, Hauber MH, Yaremko L, Britton C, Mclawhon RW, Harris AA. Pseudomembranous tracheobronchitis caused by aspergillus. *Am Rev Respir Dis* 1991;**143**:1408–11.

Keating MR, Guerrero MA, Daly RC, Walker RC, Davies SF. Transmission of invasive aspergillosis from a subclinically infected donor to three different organ transplant recipients. *Chest* 1996; **109**:1119–24.

Kramer MR, Denning DW, Marshall SE *et al*. Ulcerative Tracheobronchitis after Lung transplantation. A new form of invasive aspergillosis. *Am Rev Respir Dis* 1991;**144**:552–6.

Myers JL, Katzenstein A-LA. Granulomatous infection mimicking bronchocentric granulomatosis. *Am J Surg Pathol* 1986;**10**:317–22.

Nash G, Irvine R, Kerschmann RL, Herndier B. Pulmonary aspergillosis in acquired immune deficiency syndrome: autopsy study of an emerging pulmonary complication of human immunodeficiency virus infection. *Hum Pathol* 1997;**28**:1268–75.

Nunley DR, Ohori NP, Grgurich WF *et al*. Pulmonary Aspergillosis in cystic fibrosis lung transplant recipients. *Chest* 1998;**114**:1321–9.

Pennington JE. *Aspergillus* lung disease. *Med Clin North Am* 1980;**64**:475–91.

Schmid RA, Boehler A, Speich R, Frey H-R, Russi EW, Weder W. Bronchial anastomotic complications following lung transplantation: still a major cause of morbidity. *Eur Respir J* 1997;**10**:2872–5.

Sharma OP, Chwogule R. Many faces of pulmonary aspergillosis. *Eur Respir J* 1998;**12**:705–15.

Shumway SJ, Hertz MI, Maynard R, Kshettry VR, Bolman RM III. Airway complications after lung and heart-lung transplantation. *Transplant Proc* 1993;**25**:1165–6.

Tazelaar HD, Baird AM, Mill M, Grimes MM, Schulman LL, Smith CR. Bronchocentric mycosis occurring in transplant recipients. *Chest* 1989;**96**:92–5.

Yousem SA. The histological spectrum of chronic necrotising forms of pulmonary aspergillosis. *Hum Pathol* 1997;**28**:650–56.

SECTION TWENTY-NINE
POLYMORPHS – A FEATURE OF INFECTION

The presence of polymorphs in transbronchial biopsies and lavages is suggestive of infection particularly in large numbers, forming microabscesses and dominating the infiltrating cellular profile. Polymorphs in acute rejection infiltrates are generally dispersed amongst mononuclear cells and in the higher grades. The commonest association is with bacterial infection or superinfection which should prompt careful microbiological correlation. The latter is much more fruitful than Gram staining of biopsies and cytologic specimens.

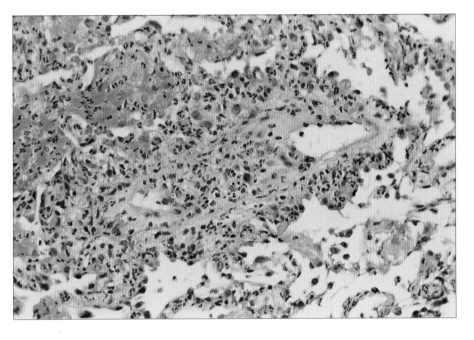

Figure 29.1

Transbronchial biopsies showing an infiltrate which is perivascular in distribution and associated with numerous polymorphs, some of which are forming small collections. Scanty eosinophils are present. The airspaces contain fibrin, macrophages and abundant polymorphs. The extension of the infiltrate into the adjacent alveolar walls is characterized by diffuse polymorph percolation into the septa. This patient had *Pseudomonas* airways infection with pneumonia and made a full response to antimicrobial therapy. The predominance of polymorphs in this infiltrate makes a diagnosis of acute rejection unlikely. Failure to respond to antibiotic therapy would be an indication for re-biopsy and assessment of any concomitant acute rejection. In a case like this, examination of the accompanying lavage which was intensely purulent, together with the results of Gram staining and culture from microbiology ensure a correct interpretation.

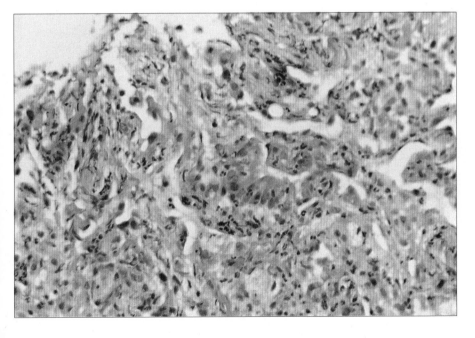

Figure 29.2

A transbronchial biopsy showing diffuse polymorph infiltration of alveolar walls with polymorphs and macrophages in alveolar spaces. There is conspicuous type II alveolar cell hyperplasia, but no evidence of viral inclusions. A small bronchiole included at the center of the field shows polymorph infiltration of the hyperplastic epithelium. Eosinophils are present but not frequent. No microabscess formation is seen. This patient grew *Pseudomonas* from airway secretions and had an intensely purulent accompanying aspirate. A full recovery was made following antimicrobial therapy.

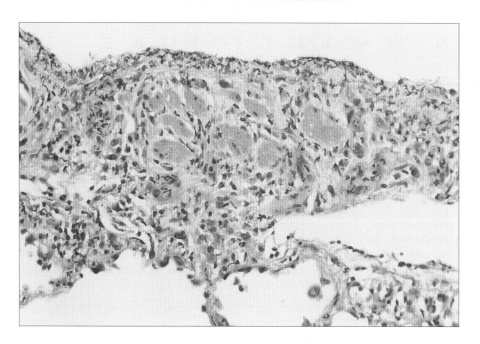

Figure 29.3

A mucosal fragment from the same biopsy shows intense infiltration by mainly polymorphs with ulceration of the epithelium. There is infiltration of inflammatory cells between the smooth muscle bundles. Type II pneumocyte hyperplasia is seen and there is extension of the inflammatory process into adjacent alveolar wall. Response was made to antipseudomonal therapy.

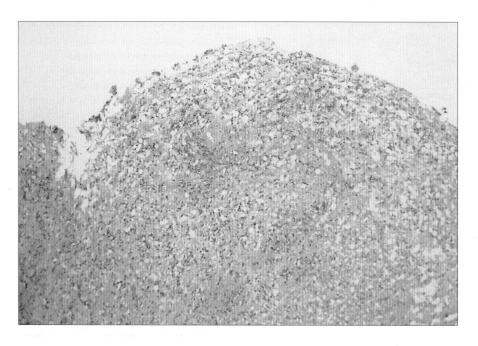

Figure 29.4

A transbronchial biopsy showing intense acute inflammation of the bronchiolar wall with effacement of normal architecture and loss of surface epithelium. The accompanying aspirate was intensely purulent with necrotic debris, culture of which gave a heavy growth of *Pseudomonas*. Antimicrobial therapy effected a full recovery. Severe ulcerative bronchiolitis in practice is much more likely to be due to common bacterial or opportunistic infection than airways rejection. A diligent search should be made for opportunistic organisms and the results of microbiological investigations awaited to make the correct diagnosis and prevent unnecessary augmented immunosuppression.

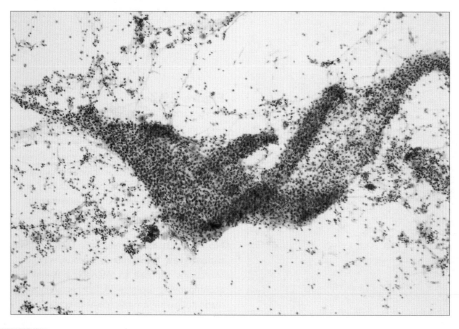

Figure 29.5

Bronchial aspirate showing frequent polymorphs in a patient with airway infection and scattered polymorphs in transbronchial biopsies. Concomitant examination of the parallel biopsies and aspirates is essential for accurate diagnosis.

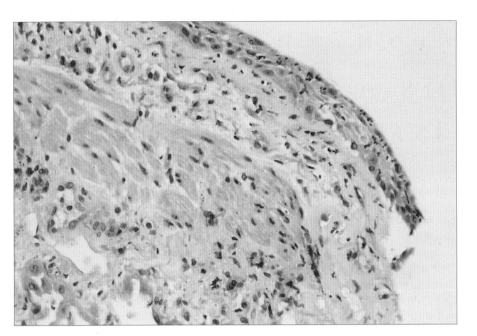

Figure 29.6
Bronchiolar surface of accompanying biopsy to Fig. 29.5 showing squamous metaplasia and epithelial infiltration by polymorphs in airway infection.

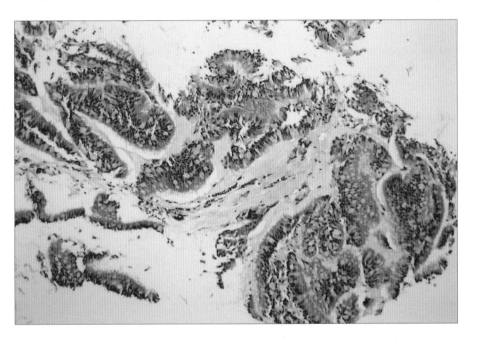

Figure 29.7
Detached fragments of bronchial epithelium with mucus and polymorphs are also strongly suggestive of airway bacterial infection and should always be carefully examined alongside parenchymal and mucosal biopsies.

FURTHER READING

Brooks RG, Hofflin JM, Jamieson SW, Stinson EB, Remington JS. Infectious complications in heart–lung recipients. *Am J Med* 1985;**79**:412–22.

Dummer SJ, Montero CG, Griffith BP, Hardesty RL, Paradis IL, Ho M. Infections in heart–lung transplant recipients. *Transplantation* 1986;**41**:725–9.

Flume P, Egan T, Paradowski L, Detterbeck F, Thompson J, Yankaskas J. Infectious complications of lung transplantation: impact of cystic fibrosis. *Am J Respir Crit Care Med* 1994;**149**:1601–7.

Ohori NP, Michaels MG, Jaffe R, Williams P, Yousem SA. Adenovirus pneumonia in lung transplant recipients. *Hum Pathol* 1995;**26**:1073–9.

Snell GI, de Hoyos A, Krajden M, Winton T, Maurer JR. *Pseudomonas cepacia* in lung transplant recipients with cystic fibrosis. *Chest* 1993;**103**:466–71.

Stockley RA. Role of bacteria in the pathogenesis and progression of acute and chronic lung infection. *Thorax* 1998;**53**:58–62.

Zenati M, Dowling RD, Dummer S *et al*. Influence of the donor lung on development of early infections in lung transplant recipients. *J Heart Transplant* 1990;**9**:502–9.

Zheng L, Orsida BE, Ward C, Wilson J W, Wiliams TJ, Walters EH, Snell GI. Airway neutrophilia in stable and bronchiolitis obliterans syndrome patients following lung transplantation. *Thorax* 2000;**55**:53–9

EOSINOPHILS – A FEATURE OF INFECTION

Infiltration of mucosa and lung parenchyma by eosinophils is a relatively common feature of lung transplant biopsies. They may be an integral part of the higher grades of acute rejection, but when they comprise more than 50% of the inflammatory infiltrate other causes are usually found. In the airway, infection by *Pseudomonas* species can be associated with a dense eosinophilic infiltrate which may induce clinical symptoms of airflow obstruction indistinguishable from asthma. If the response to antimicrobial therapy is incomplete these patients often respond well to inhaled steroid treatment. It is important to recognize though that steroids in this circumstance are not being administered to treat acute rejection by augmenting immunosuppression. Another important cause of eosinophil infiltration in both airways and parenchyma is fungal infection, most commonly by *Aspergillus*, and an intense reaction can be mounted to a relatively low fungal load. Again, in close collaboration with microbiological findings a good response may be obtained by adding inhaled or systemic steroids to antifungal

treatment. Eosinophils are well-described in pulmonary drug reactions, e.g. nitrofurantoin, sulphasalazine, penicillin. In the setting of lung transplant recipients there are many potential causes and it is exceedingly difficult to ascribe an eosinophilic infiltrate to a specific drug, but in the absence of other identifiable causes and failure to respond to treatment removal of the suspected drug may be beneficial.

It is possible to stain immunohistochemically for markers of eosinophil activation. This has mainly been used in research on biopsies. In clinical practice however, it is useful to recognize degranulating eosinophils in a biopsy as this generally indicates a need for treatment. Abundant eosinophils with degranulation can be recognized in the accompanying bronchial aspirate in cases with significant eosinophil infiltration of biopsies. In our practice of staining aspirates with hematoxylin and eosin, the eosinophils are readily recognized and no further special stains are required for their identification.

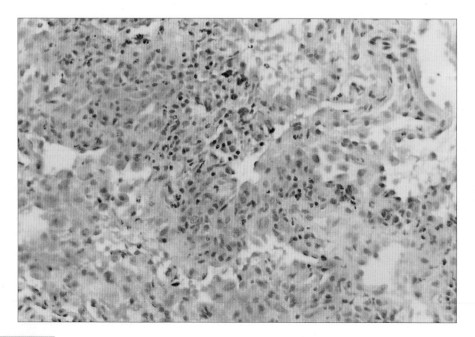

Figure 30.1
Transbronchial biopsy showing a high-power view of a perivascular infiltrate in which there are significant numbers of eosinophils. There is involvement of alveolar walls and spaces indicating that this is an A3 rejection in which this proportion of eosinophils in the infiltrate is well-recognized. Infection should as always be carefully excluded to avoid missing a mixed rejection and infection picture, the most likely organisms being *Pseudomonas* or *Aspergillus*. In this case no infection was diagnosed and the patient recovered on increased immunosuppression.

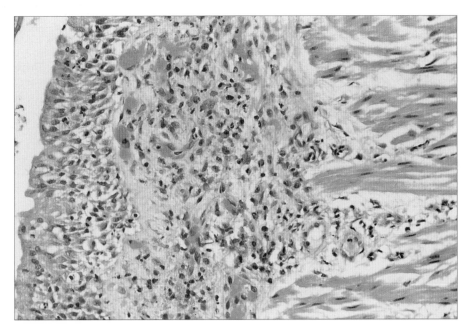

Figure 30.2
The bronchial biopsy submitted with a set of transbronchial biopsies shows intense subepithelial eosinophil infiltration with infiltration of the hyperplastic overlying epithelium by eosinophils also. There is evidence of degranulation with eosinophilic granules in the lamina propria extracellularly. Polymorphs are also present but are not the predominant inflammatory cells. This patient grew abundant *Pseudomonas* and had an intensely purulent appearance to the airways at bronchoscopy and to the accompanying aspirate. Eosinophilic inflammation in the airways and *Pseudomonas* infection is well-recognized in lung allografts and should not be confused with airways acute rejection.

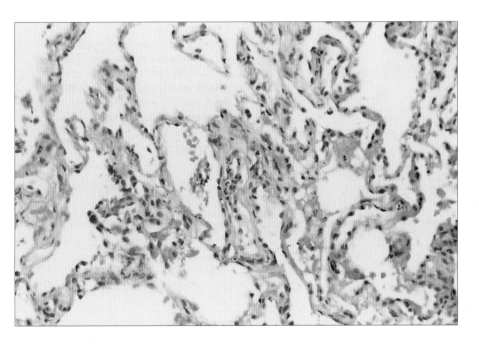

Figure 30.3
Transbronchial parenchymal fragments from the same biopsy as Fig. 30.2 show infiltration of the alveolar walls by polymorphs and eosinophils. No perivascular infiltrates were present in any of the biopsy fragments. The interstitial eosinophils in these cases are usually less dense and numerous than in the airways. Interstitial eosinophils in the presence of normal airways or in biopsy series without airways included should alert the pathologist and clinician to the possibility of infection.

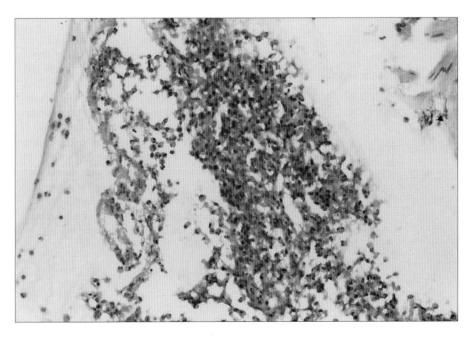

Figure 30.4
Biopsy series occasionally include sheets of eosinophils and macrophages with mucus as detached fragments. This appearance is most frequently associated with *Aspergillus* infection and can occur in the presence of normal parenchyma. This patient grew *Aspergillus* from the accompanying lavage and developed bronchiectasis with bronchocentric granulomatous mycosis for which a transplant lobectomy was required. The fungal elements in such cases may be very sparse and not identified histologically or cytologically.

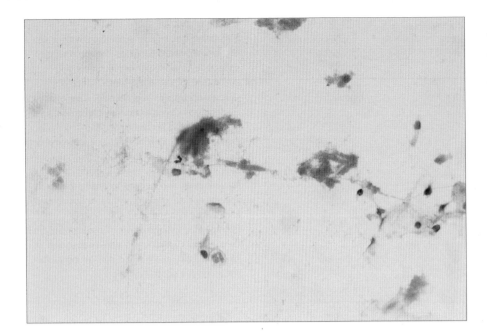

Figure 30.5
The accompanying lavage of Fig. 30.4 showed eosinophils and Charcot–Leyden crystals derived from the eosinophils. These are easily recognized on a hemotoxylin and eosin-stained smear of the aspirate as sharp-ended needle-like crystals.

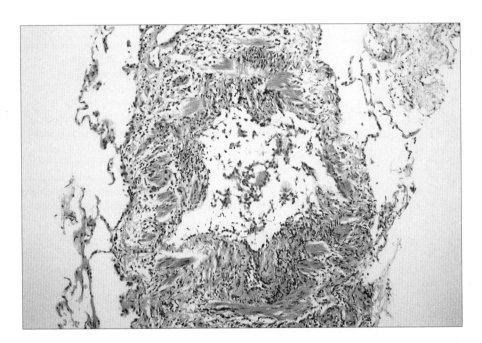

Figure 30.6
Transbronchial biopsy including a bronchiole with a loose but definite circumferential infiltrate on both sides of the airway smooth muscle including frequent eosinophils. The lumen contains desquamated epithelial cells.

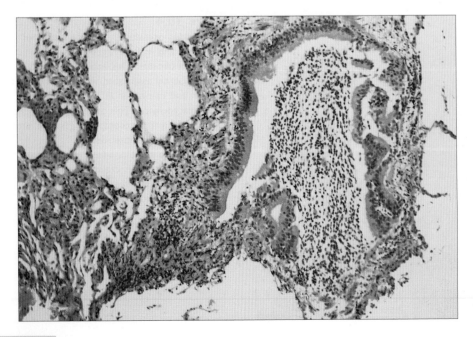

Figure 30.7
Higher power view of the airway in Fig. 30.6 shows numerous eosinophils in the infiltrate breaching the smooth muscle and associated with edema. Another bronchiole in the same biopsy shows eosinophils and mucus accumulated within the bronchiolar lumen. The bronchiolar epithelium itself shows minimal infiltration only. The adjacent parenchyma shows non-specific features of hemosiderin-laden macrophages and minor alveolar wall infiltration. Numerous Charcot–Leyden crystals and eosinophils were present in the accompanying lavage and cultures grew *Pseudomonas* and *Aspergillus*.

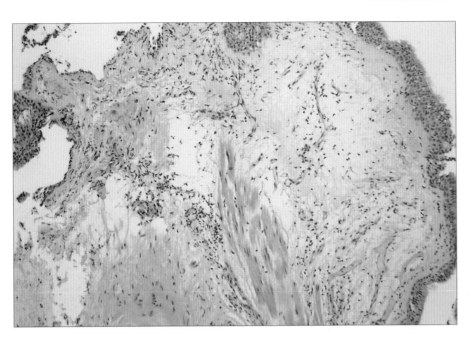

Figure 30.8
Transbronchial biopsy in which the airway shows marked edema but not fibrosis. There is a mild inflammatory infiltrate with frequent eosinophils. This patient had new deterioration of function in the setting of obliterative bronchiolitis due to Pseudomonal airway infection.

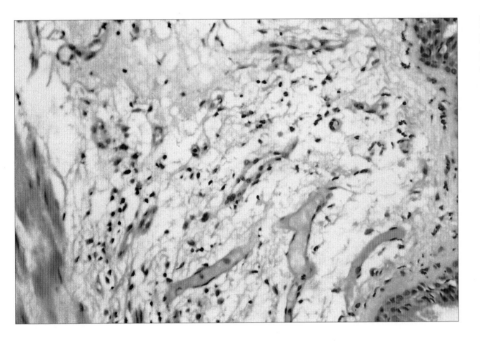

Figure 30.9
High-power view of edematous lamina propria with eosinophils some of which are degranulated.

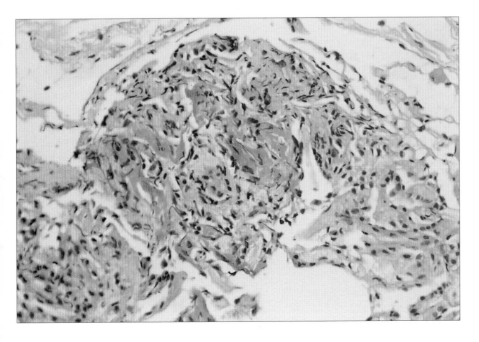

Figure 30.10
The parenchymal sample of the same biopsy shows some organization of fibrin with both eosinophils and polymorphs. These inflammatory cells frequently co-exist in lung transplant biopsies in the presence of infection.

FURTHER READING

Dosanjh AK, Elashoff D, Kawalek A, Moss RB, Esrig S. Activation of eosinophils in the airways of lung transplant patients. *Chest* 1997;**112**:1180–83.

Dosanjh AK, Robinson TE, Strauss J, Berry G. Eosinophil activation in cardiac and pulmonary acute allograft rejection. *J Heart Lung Transplant* 1999;**17**:1038.

Maurer JR, Tullis E, Grossman RF, Velland H, Winton TL, Patterson GA. Infectious complications following isolated lung transplantation. *Chest* 1992;**101**:1056–9.

Yousem SA. Graft eosinophilia in lung transplantation. *Hum Pathol* 1992;**23**:1172–7.

SECTION THIRTY-ONE

POST-TRANSPLANT
LYMPHOPROLIFERATIVE DISEASE

Post-transplant lymphoproliferative disease is seen more commonly in lung transplant than heart transplant recipients which is probably due to the higher level of immunosuppression. It is most often B-cell in type and related to Epstein–Barr virus (EBV infection). Unlike other solid organ recipients the lung itself is a common site for the presentation of disease which is an important differential diagnosis of new nodules on chest X-ray and CT. Diagnosis can be made by transbronchial biopsy or by needle aspiration and cutting needle biopsies, alternatively the diagnosis being made on nodal tissue or from another extranodal site. Post-transplant lymphoproliferative disease may also be an unsuspected diagnosis at autopsy due to lack of specificity of clinical presentation.

Post-transplant lymphoproliferative disease (PTLPD) in the lung shows diffuse sheet-like infiltration with neoplastic lymphoid cells and foci of coagulative necrosis. Angioinvasion with or without fibrinoid necrosis may be seen and this together with the diffuse nature of the infiltrate with necrosis allows distinction from severe acute pulmonary rejection. Morphologically the lymphoproliferation may be of pleomorphic or monomorphic type and can be classified into low- and high-grade types. Immunohistochemical and molecular methods may further refine the diagnosis. It is however not possible to predict from the biopsy appearances the response to therapy. Apparently high-grade PTLPD may regress with decreased immunosuppression and antiviral therapy, but chemotherapy may be required in patients with aggressive clinical disease of higher stage.

There have been many classifications of PTLPD encompassing the diversity of clinical, histopathologic, immunologic and genotypic features (Table 10). A recent working classification has been proposed to include all recognized types in a single scheme but this is outside the scope of lung biopsies, often requiring nodal tissue for diagnosis (Table 11). In practise, PTLPD in the grafted lung tends to be of high-grade, falling into the polymorphic B-cell categories or monomorphic if a majority of neoplastic cells are transformed. The growth pattern of these types is tumorous with invasion and destruction allowing separation from benign or reactive differential diagnoses. These PTLPDs have varying clonal predominance and it seems that those with the smaller clonal populations are most likely to make a response to decreased immunosuppression. Once diagnosed with PTLPD, it is essential to refer the lung allograft recipient to an oncologist with specialist expertise in this area for full staging and work-up so that the most appropriate treatment of decreased immunosuppression or chemotherapy can be administered.

The diagnosis of PTLPD can be elusive and it has been significantly under-recognized in life with the diagnosis only being made at autopsy. The various appearances in the lung are therefore illustrated at length in this section.

Table 10

Post-transplantation lymphoproliferative disorders: Classification by Knowles et al.

Plasmacytic hyperplastia
Polymorphic PTLPD (polymorphic B-cell hyperplasia and polymorphic B-cell lymphoma)
Immunoblastic lymphoma/multiple myeloma

From: Knowles DM, Cesarman E, Chadburn A, Frizzera G, Chen J, Rose EA, Michler RE. *Blood* 1995;**85**:552–65.

Table 11

A working classification of lymphoproliferative lesions in transplant patients

Plasmacytic hyperplasia	PH
Post-transplant lymphoproliferative disorders	PTLD
Infectious mononucleosis-like	IM–PTLD
Plasma cell rich	PC–PTLD
Polymorphic	P–PTLD
Monomorphic	M–PTLD
Multiple myeloma-like	MM–PTLD
T-cell type	T–PTLD
Hodgkin's disease-like	HD–PTLD
Composite	C–PTLD
Not otherwise specified	PTLD–NOS
Other	

From: Swerdlow SH. *Curr Diagn Pathol* 1997;**4**:28–35.

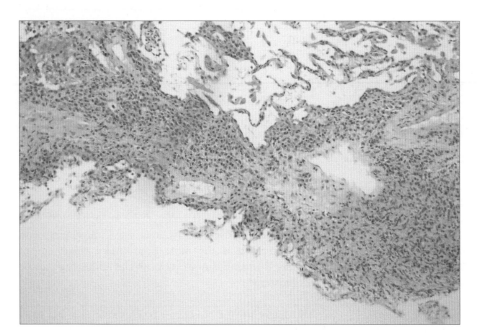

Figure 31.1
Transbronchial biopsy at low-power showing sheet like infiltration centered on a vessel which extends into nodular conformation where it infiltrates parenchyma. There is some minor involvement of adjacent alveolar walls at low-power and a small vessel in parenchyma is also cuffed. The infiltrate is densely cellular and uniform. No endothelialitis is seen.

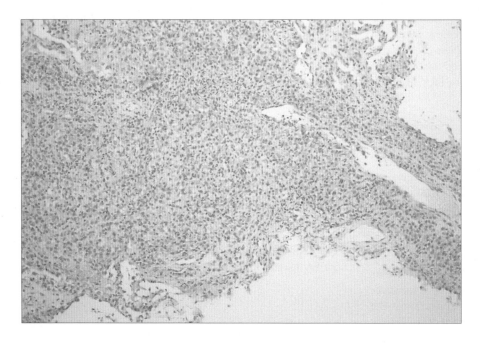

Figure 31.2
Higher power showing the diffuse sheet-like nature of the infiltrates in the same biopsy which in this field involves the full thickness of the vessel wall including endothelium. The diffuse nature of the mononuclear infiltrate forming a solid sheet of tumor is strikingly different from the infiltrates of high-grade rejection both qualitatively and quantitatively. The formation of a mass lesion with infiltration and destruction of lung tissue differentiates PTLPD from benign, reactive conditions.

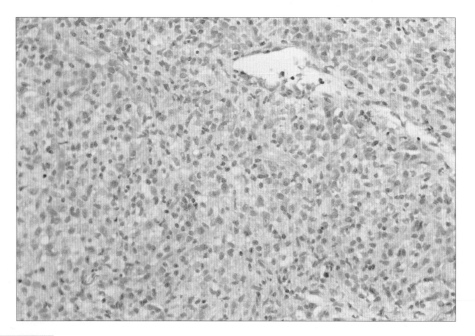

Figure 31.3
Same infiltrate at high-power showing sheet-like mainly large lymphocytes with moderate cytoplasm and prominent nucleoli. Involvement of the endothelium with these neoplastic lymphoid cells is clearly seen. There is no evidence of necrosis in this patients infiltrate. At this power the plasmacytoid appearance of some of the cells is evident. This has the features of a polymorphic B-cell PTLPD.

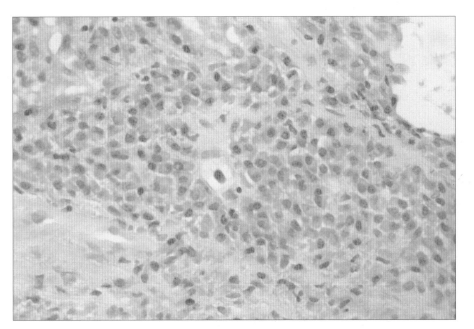

Figure 31.4
Another field in the same biopsy fragment shows the plasmacytoid features more clearly with eccentric nuclei and eosinophilic cytoplasm. The monotony of the infiltrate and the cytologic abnormality of the cells including those in the endothelium allows distinction from rejection even in small biopsy samples.

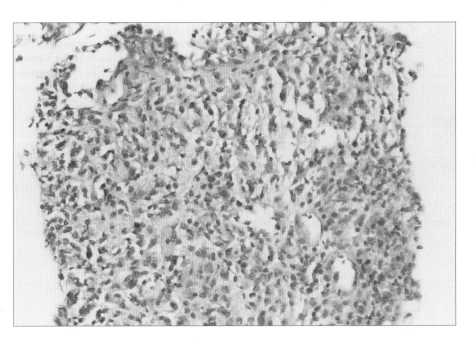

Figure 31.5
Transbronchial biopsy from another patient showing lymphoproliferative disease diffusely infiltrating the lung tissue with effacement of normal architecture. The predominance of large atypical lymphoid cells is seen with few mature small lymphocytes in the background. The main differential diagnosis is acute rejection which at this degree of cellularity would be expected to show polymorphs, eosinophils and macrophages. The cytologic and architectural features however point to the correct diagnosis of PTLPD. This patient had disseminated lymphoproliferative disease at autopsy.

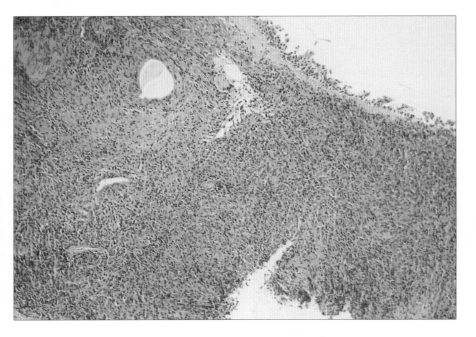

Figure 31.6
Transbronchial biopsy from a patient with an unsuspected odd bronchoscopic appearance. This endobronchial biopsy fragment shows diffuse infiltration by cellular neoplasm with sparing of the basement membrane and epithelium. The sheet-like diffuse nature is typical of lymphoproliferative disease. There is no non-neoplastic condition in the transplanted airway which shows this degree of monotonous cellular infiltration. This appearance can be distinguished from exuberant bronchus-associated lymphoid tissue by the lack of follicular, vascular and organoid structure.

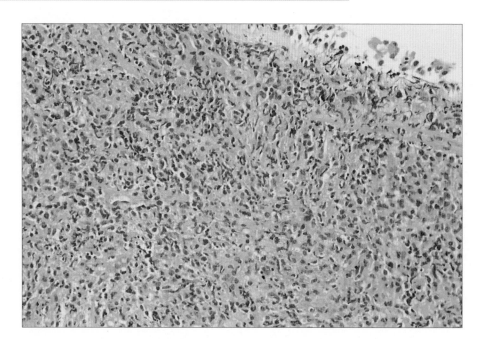

Figure 31.7
Higher power of the same biopsy shows the neoplastic lymphoid infiltrate with some conspicuously enlarged hyperchromatic cells and involvement of the surface epithelium in this field. The appearances at this power are of a high-grade lymphoproliferative disorder most in keeping with polymorphic B-cell PTLPD but monomorphic B-cell PTLPD, which is usually monoclonal cannot be excluded on this histologic appearance.

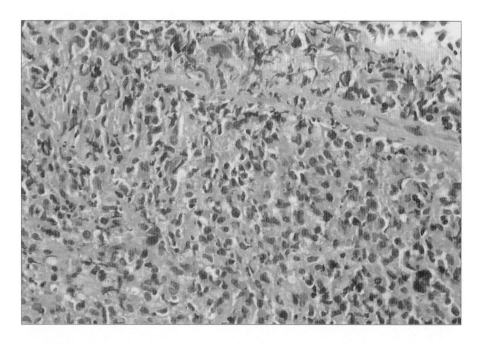

Figure 31.8
The preponderance of large atypical lymphoid cells is clearly seen at the highest power with infiltration across the muscularis at the top of the field. Mitoses are seen but there is no evidence of necrosis in this airway infiltrate. In small biopsy samples it is difficult to distinguish polymorphic from monomorphic PTLPD. Pleomorphic PTLPD is best classified as monomorphic but the variability from field to field is a problem with small tissue biopsies.

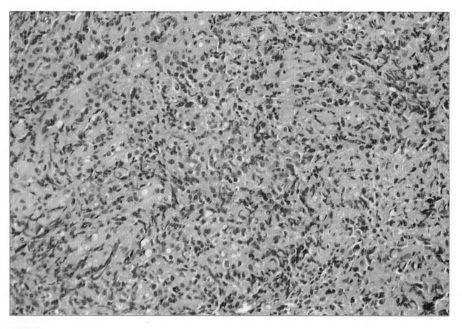

Figure 31.9
Deep in the endobronchial sample adjacent to peribronchiolar parenchyma there is an extension of the lymphoproliferation. Same case as Fig. 31.6.

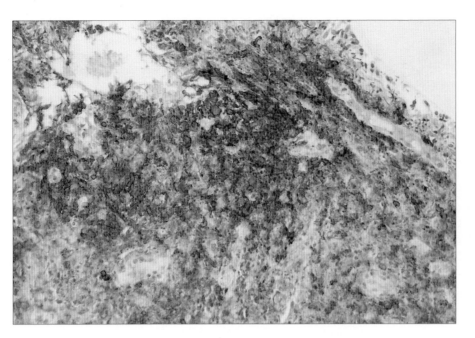

Figure 31.10
The bronchial infiltrate is strongly CD20 positive confirming the B-cell nature of the neoplastic population. Acute rejection infiltrates are dominated by T-cells in comparison.

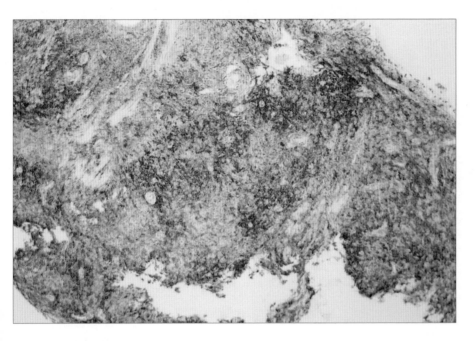

Figure 31.11
A faint nodularity to the infiltrate is revealed by CD20 staining where the lymphoproliferation abuts parenchyma.

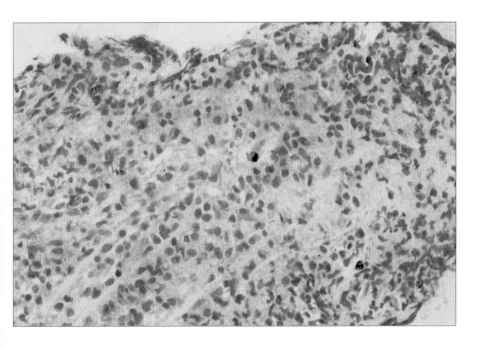

Figure 31.12
Scattered cells in the infiltrate stain strongly with Epstein–Barr virus LMP1 (latent membrane protein 1).

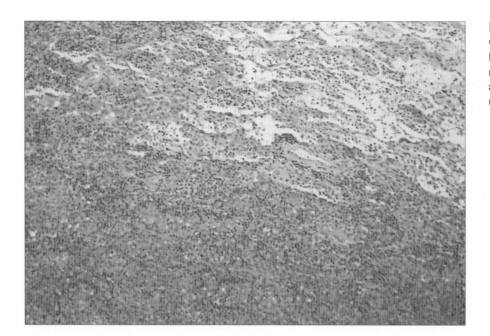

Figure 31.13
Open lung biopsy showing lymphoproliferative disease forming a large nodule which was visible radiographically and infiltration of alveolar walls at its margin.

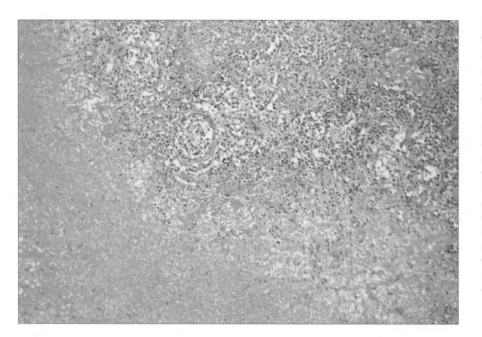

Figure 31.14
Within the nodule there are large areas of coagulative necrosis. This pattern of necrosis is uncommon in other post-transplant pathologies. On small biopsy fragments coagulative necrosis should always raise a high index of suspicion of lymphoproliferative disease. At the margins of the necrotic area the neoplastic lymphoid infiltrate involves the full thickness of a vessel wall with occlusion of its lumen. The high-grade nature of the infiltrate is clearly seen with many large atypical lymphoid cells and numerous mitoses. In the center of the nodule on the open biopsy the anaplastic nature of the infiltrate in this case is seen with frequent mitotic figures and large immunoblasts. The patient died despite therapy. Monomorphic B-cell PTLPD.

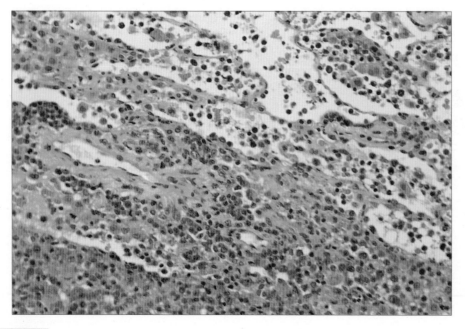

Figure 31.15
High-power view of the margin of the nodule with normal parenchyma shows pattern of infiltration characteristic of lymphoid neoplasms in the lung. The cytologic features of the cells should alert the pathologist to the neoplastic nature of this process even on small biopsy fragments.

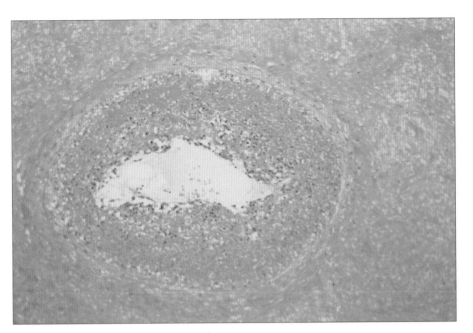

Figure 31.16

The center of the nodule shows full thickness fibrinoid necrosis of a large vessel with neoplastic infiltration of its wall including the endothelium. The atypical nature of the infiltrate clearly distinguishes it from acute rejection which very rarely at its highest grade shows fibrinoid vasculitis in open biopsy or autopsy material. The tendency to involve vessels explains the high incidence of necrosis in high-grade PTLPD in the lung.

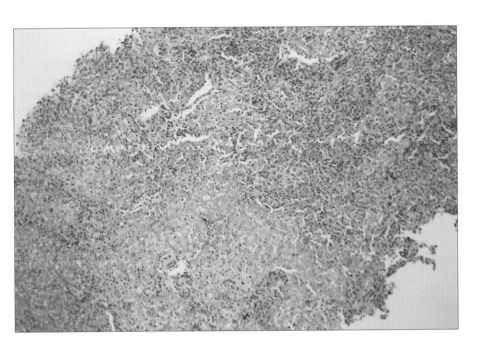

Figure 31.17

Transbronchial biopsy fragment with both necrotic and viable lymphoproliferative disease. The pattern of necrosis is a very useful pointer to the correct diagnosis in cases which are less cytologically neoplastic.

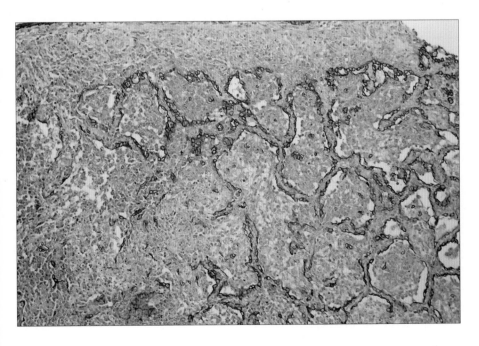

Figure 31.18

AE1/AE3 staining of a nodule of lymphoproliferative disease highlighting the diffuse nature of the infiltrate with preservation of alveolar architecture not evident on H & E staining. Elsewhere there was destruction with parenchymal necrosis.

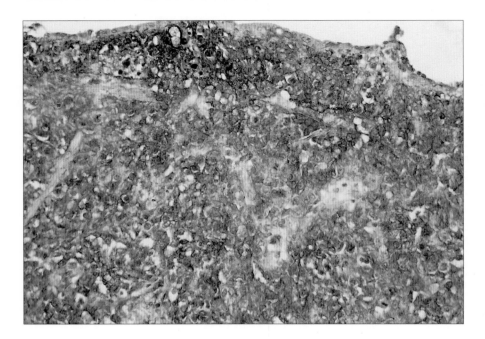

Figure 31.19
CD20 immunostaining of an open lung biopsy involved in post-transplant lymphoproliferative disease. The neoplastic infiltrates are very commonly almost exclusively B-cell in nature as shown here. T-cell and Hodgkin's-like PTLPD have however been reported in lung allograft recipients.

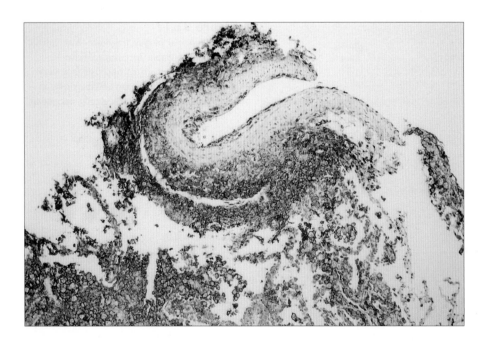

Figure 31.20
Transbronchial biopsy showing lymphoproliferative disease highlighted with leukocyte common antigen (LCA) staining. The sheet-like infiltrate is perivascular with involvement of the endothelium but sparing of the media.

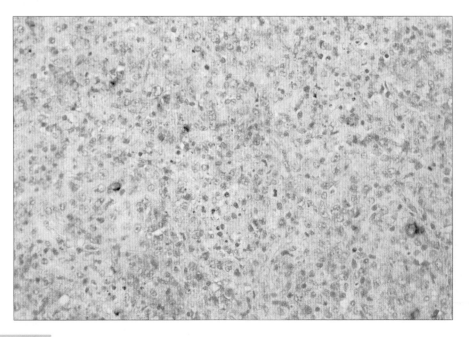

Figure 31.21
Immunohistochemical staining for Epstein–Barr virus in open lung biopsy taken for diagnosis of new chest X-ray nodules. Positive atypical cells are demonstrated with LMP-1 antibody on immunoperoxidase staining.

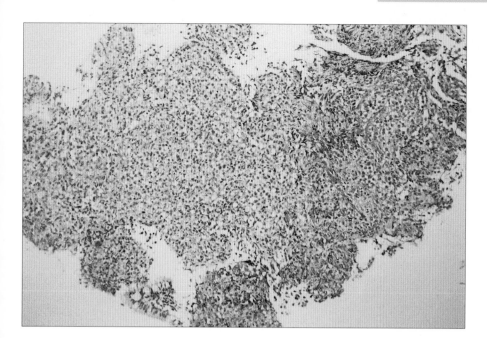

Figure 31.22
Necrotic fragment of transbronchial biopsy in patient with new nodules on chest X-ray. The fragment shows coagulative necrosis with some viable cells. This biopsy appearance is common in lymphoproliferative disease in the transplanted lung. Diagnosis can be made on core biopsies with adequate gauge needles. Aspiration or screw biopsies for cytologic assessment alone are not recommended for initial diagnosis but may be adequate for recurrent disease.

FURTHER READING

Aris RM, Maia DM, Neuringer IP *et al.* Post-transplantation lymphoproliferative disorder in the Epstein–Barr virus-naive lung transplant recipient. *Am J Respir Crit Care Med* 1996;**154**:1712–17.

Berg LC, Copenhaver CM, Morrison VA *et al.* B-cell lymphoproliferative disorders in solid organ transplant patients: Detection of Epstein–Barr virus by *in situ* hybridization. *Hum Pathol* 1992;**23**:159–63.

Carbone A, Dolcetti R, Gloghini A *et al.* Immunophenotypic and molecular analyses of acquired immune deficiency syndrome – related and Epstein–Barr virus-associated lymphomas. A comparative study. *Hum Pathol* 1996;**27**:133–46.

Chetty R, Biddolph S, Gatter K. An immunohistochemical analysis of Reed–Sternberg-like cells in posttransplantation lymphoproliferative disorders: The possible pathogenetic relationship to Reed–Sternberg cells in Hodgkin's disease and Reed–Sternberg-like cells in non-Hodgkin's lymphomas and reactive conditions. *Hum Pathol* 1997;**28**:493–8.

Chetty R, Biddolph S, Kaklamanis L, Cary N, Stewart S, Giatromanolaki A, Gatter K. bcl-2 protein is strongly expressed in post-transplant lymphoproliferative disorders. *J Pathol* 1996;**180**:254–8.

Egan JJ, Hasleton PS, Yonan N *et al.* Necrotic, ulcerative bronchitis, the presenting feature of lymphoproliferative disease following heart–lung transplantation. *Thorax* 1995;**50**:205–7.

Frizerra G, Hanto DW, Gajl-Peczalska KJ *et al.* Polymorphic diffuse B-cell hyperplasia and lymphomas in renal transplant recipients. *Cancer Res* 1981;**41**:4262–79.

Goldman M, Gérard C, Abramowicz D *et al.* Induction of interleukin-6 and interleukin-10 by the OKT3 monoclonal antibody: Possible relevance to post transplant lymphoproliferative disorders. *Clin Transplant* 1992;**6**:265–8.

Hanto DW. Polyclonal and monoclonal post transplant lymphoproliferative disease (LPD). *Clin Transplant* 1992;**6**:227–34.

Knowles DM, Cesarman E, Chadburn A *et al.* Correlative morphologic and molecular genetic analysis demonstrates three distinct categories of posttransplantation lymphoproliferative disorders. *Blood* 1995;**85**:552–65.

Levine SM, Angel L, Anzueto A *et al.* A low incidence of posttransplant lymphoproliferative disorder in 109 lung transplant recipients. *Chest* 1999;**116**:1273–7.

Lones MA, Shintaku IP, Weiss LM, Thung SN, Nichols WS, Geller SA. Posttransplant lymphoproliferative disorder in liver allograft biopsies: a comparison of three methods for the demonstration of Epstein–Barr virus. *Hum Pathol* 1997;**28**:533–9.

Nalesnik MA, Jaffe R, Starzl TE *et al.* The pathology of post-transplant lymphoproliferative disorders occurring in the setting of cyclosporin A prednisolone immunosuppression. *Am J Pathol* 1988;**133**:173–92.

Nalesnik MA, Locker J, Jaffe R *et al.* Experience with posttransplant lymphoproliferative disorders in solid organ transplant recipients. *Clin Transplant* 1992;**6**:249–52.

Nalesnik MA. Post transplantation lymphoproliferative disorders (PTLD): Current perspectives. *Sem Thorac Cardiovasc Surg.* 1996;**8**:139–48.

Randhawa PS, Yousem SA, Paradis IL, Dauber JA, Griffith BP, Locker J. The clinical spectrum, pathology and clonal analysis of Epstein-Barr virus associated lymphoproliferative disorders in heart-lung transplant recipients. *Am J Clin Path* 1989;**92**:177–85.

Randhawa S, Yousem SA. Epstein–Barr virus-associated lymphoproliferative disease in a heart-lung allograft. *Transplantation* 1990;**49**:126–30.

Rosendale B, Yousem SA. Discrimination of Epstein–Barr virus-related post transplant lymphoproliferations from acute rejection in lung allograft recipients. *Arch Pathol Lab Med* 1995;**119**:48–423.

Swerdlow SH. Post-transplant lymphoproliferative disorders: a working classification. *Curr Diagnost Pathol* 1997;**4**:28–35.

Swerdlow S. Post-transplant lymphoproliferative disorders: a morphologic, phenotypic and genotypic spectrum of disease. *Histopathology* 1992;**20**:373–85.

Wu T-T, Swerdlow SH, Locker J *et al*. Recurrent Epstein–Barr virus-associated lesions in organ transplant recipients. *Hum Pathol* 1996;**27**:157–64.

Yousem SA, Randhawa P, Locker J *et al*. Post transplant lymphoproliferative disorders in heart lung transplant recipients: primary presentation in the allograft. *Hum Pathol* 1989;**20**:361–9.

Histopathologic features of diffuse alveolar damage may occasionally be seen in biopsies from lung transplants. The histopathologic changes are the same as in native lungs, with acute exudate, subacute proliferative and chronic fibrous phases recognized. There are hyaline membranes lining alveolar spaces in the acute phase with interstitial widening and a mild inflammatory cell infiltrate. As the process evolves there is organization with a more pronounced inflammatory infiltrate, proliferation of fibroblasts and granulation tissue formation. There is often prominent pneumocyte hyperplasia with enlarged nuclei and often prominent nucleoli, which can be mistaken for viral inclusions.

In the transplant setting the differential diagnosis includes severe ischemia-reperfusion injury and severe acute rejection and close clinical correlation is needed. As with the general population other causes include infection either viral or associated with systemic sepsis, hemorrhage, aspiration and oxygen and ventilatory therapy.

Diffuse alveolar damage may therefore be the biopsy or autopsy pathologic appearance in primary graft failure which is an ischemic/reperfusion injury with non-cardiogenic pulmonary edema. Some cases are mild and self-limiting but others, a minority, develop severe persistent graft dysfunction with a requirement for prolonged ventilation. Primary graft failure is therefore a diagnosis of exclusion after pneumonia, aspiration, fluid overload, pulmonary venous anastomotic complication and acute rejection have been excluded.

Concomitant acute rejection may also be seen in diffuse alveolar damage but cannot be graded in the presence of other changes. Diffuse alveolar damage as a *result* of acute rejection occurs only in Grade A4. Concomitant infection such as bronchopneumonia is also likely to be secondary to the initial ischemic insult or donor-related. The donor history is important in early diffuse alveolar damage.

Hyperacute rejection is very rare indeed and described at autopsy rather than on transbronchial biopsies as it occurs as soon as the graft is implanted. It shows features of diffuse microvascular thrombi formation with alveolar wall infiltration by neutrophils rather than diffuse alveolar damage.

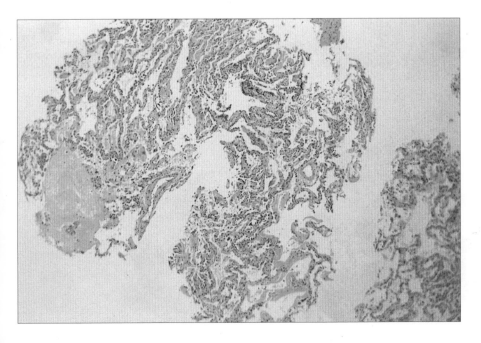

Figure 32.1
Transbronchial biopsy at low-power showing alveolar wall thickening due to inflammatory cells with fibrin and hemorrhage. No perivascular infiltrates are discernible at low-power. This patient showed worsening of lung function and chest X-ray shadowing at 4 days having done well initially postoperatively.

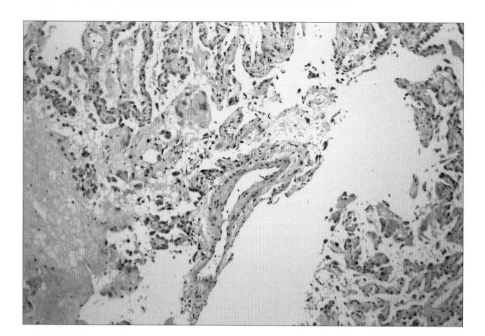

Figure 32.2
Higher power view of the biopsy confirms interstitial inflammation with fibrin. The lack of perivascular distribution to the infiltrate is clearly shown. There is type II cell hyperplasia and the pathologic process appears diffuse and acute in nature.

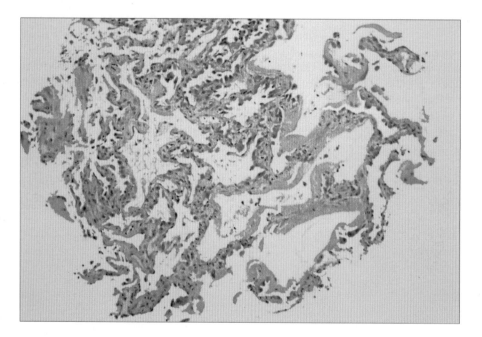

Figure 32.3
Elsewhere in the biopsy hyaline membranes confirm the diagnosis of diffuse alveolar damage. It is relatively uncommon to perform transbronchial biopsies at 4 days so the 'baseline' appearances are unknown. Adequate samples with a clear diagnosis of diffuse alveolar damage can obviate the need for open lung biopsy. In this case the cause was ascribed to donor infection but an additional effect of reperfusion injury cannot be absolutely excluded. The patient made a full recovery.

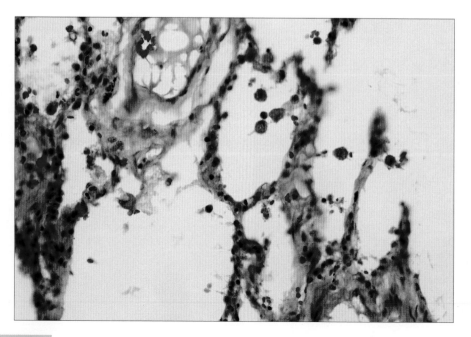

Figure 32.4
High-power view of an unused partner donor lung with fat emboli from long bone fractures prior to brain death.

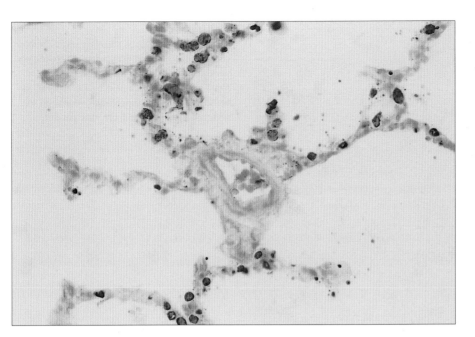

Figure 32.5
The presence of globules of fat in the capillaries is confirmed by oil red O staining. Donors with fractures need to be carefully evaluated in view of the risk of fat or bone marrow embolism.

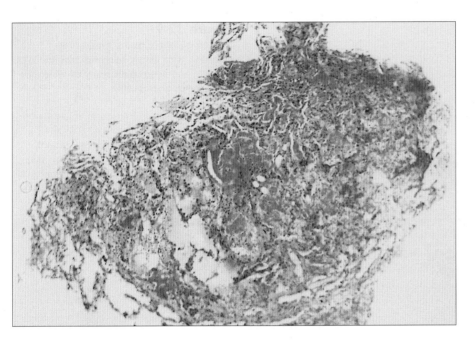

Figure 32.6
Low-power view of transbronchial biopsy from recipient of the partner donor lung of Fig. 32.4 showing pneumonic consolidation with conspicuous fibrin. The patient had radiologic opacification of the lung shortly after transplantation and early transbronchial biopsy was performed.

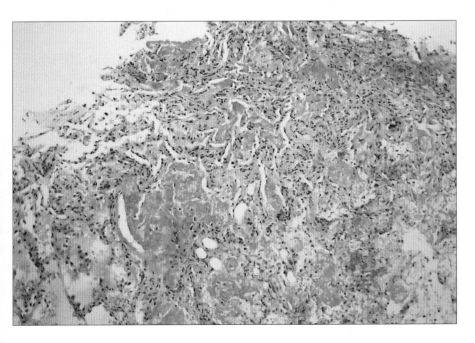

Figure 32.7
High-power view of the transbronchial biopsy confirms the consolidation due to fibrinous pneumonia. No hyaline membranes were present. The patient recovered with careful fluid restriction and the dysfunction in the newly grafted lung was attributed to fat emboli in the donor. This probably occurs to a lesser extent in many transplanted lungs, but highlights the importance of considering factors in the donor when dealing with the very early postoperative transbronchial biopsies.

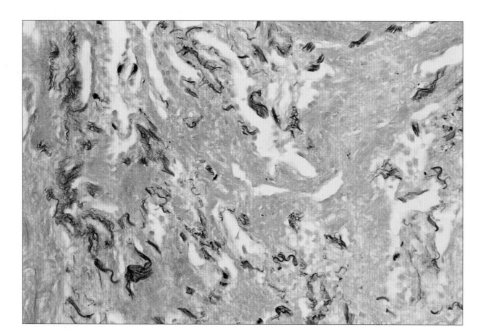

Figure 32.8
Transbronchial biopsy showing intra-alveolar fibrosis and hemosiderin-laden macrophages several months after acute respiratory distress syndrome caused by perioperative hemorrhage. This appearance was seen in several later biopsies from this patient.

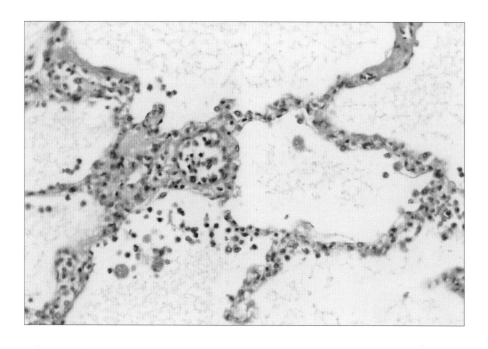

Figure 32.9
Section of lung showing hyperacute rejection with diffuse microvascular thrombi of fibrin and neutrophils many of which are adherent to endothelium.

FURTHER READING

Bridges ND, Spray TL, Collins MH, Bowles NE, Towbin JA. Adenovirus infection in the lung results in graft failure after lung transplantation. *J Thorac Cardiovasc Surg* 1998;**116**:617–23.

Chaparro C, Chamberlain D, Maurer J, De Hoyos A, Winton T, Kesten S. Acute lung injury in lung allografts. *J Heart Lung Transplant* 1995; **14**:267–73.

Choi JK, Kearns J, Palevsky HI *et al*. Hyperacute rejection of a pulmonary allograft. Immediate clinical and pathological findings. *Am J Respir Crit Care Med* 1999;**160**:1015–18.

Christie JD, Bavaria JE, Palevsky HI *et al*. Primary graft failure following lung transplantation. *Chest* 1998;**114**:51–60.

Egan TM, Boychuk JE, Rosato K, Cooper JD. Whence the lungs? A study to assess suitability of donor lungs for transplantation. *Transplantation* 1992; **53**:420–2.

Frost AE, Jammal CT, Cagle PT. Hyperacute rejection following lung transplantation. *Chest* 1996;**110**:559–62.

Paradis IL, Duncan SR, Dauber JH, Yousem S, Hardesty R, Griffith B. Distinguishing between infection, rejection and the adult respiratory distress syndrome after human lung transplantation. *J Heart Lung Transplant* 1992;**11**:S232–6.

Pham S M, Yoshida Y, Aeba R *et al*. Interleukin-6, a marker of preservation injury in clinical lung transplantation. *J Heart Lung Transplant* 1992; **11**:1017–24.

Schulman LL. Perioperative mortality and primary graft failure. *Chest* 1998;**114**:7–8.

Sleiman C, Mal H, Fourner M *et al.* Pulmonary reimplantation response in single-lung transplantation. *Eur Respir J* 1995;8:5–9.

Sommers KE, Griffiths BP, Hardesty RL, Keenan RJ. Early lung allograft function in twin recipients from the same donor: Risk factor analysis. *Ann Thorac Surg* 1996;**62**:784–90.

Zenati M, Yousem SA, Dowling RD, Stein KL, Griffith BP. Primary graft failure following pulmonary transplantation. *Transplantation* 1990;**50**:165–7.

RECURRENT DISEASE

The etiology of many of the conditions for which lungs are transplanted is not known and with increasing length of survival post-transplantation, it is clear that some conditions recur in the graft in the presence of immunosuppression. This phenomenon of recurrence is of great biological interest for understanding pathogenesis of the conditions in view of the new host milieu. It also poses diagnostic problems in the graft and further widens the differential diagnoses to be considered in post-transplant biopsies. It is wise to report biopsies in full knowledge of the primary diagnosis leading to transplantation. The most likely conditions to recur are sarcoidosis, Langerhans' cell histiocytosis, lymphangioleiomyomatosis, desquamative interstitial pneumonia and giant cell interstitial pneumonia according to experience from larger centers. Before accepting granulomas in biopsies as being due to recurrent sarcoidosis, opportunistic infection should be carefully excluded. The impact of recurrence on survival is difficult to assess due to relatively small numbers, but sarcoidosis does not have major impact. Failure to stop smoking may increase the likelihood of recurrence of smoking-related conditions such as Langerhans' cell histiocytosis and desquamative interstitial pneumonitis.

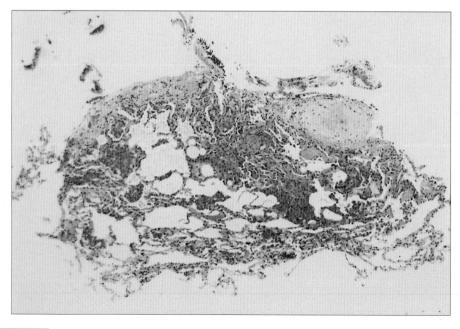

Figure 33.1
Transbronchial biopsy from a patient transplanted for sarcoidosis of the heart and lungs. At low-power, non-caseating epithelioid granulomata are clearly seen in the parenchyma with are discrete and not associated with other interstitial inflammation. Opportunist infection was meticulously excluded and cultures of biopsy and accompanying lavage were negative. The appearances are those of recurrent sarcoidosis in the graft. This recurrence is generally without clinical significance but poses potential problems in biopsy interpretation.

Figure 33.2
Low-power transbronchial biopsy with a fragment of bronchial cartilage and parenchyma showing filling of alveolar spaces by cells which appear faintly pigmented. The patient had been transplanted a few weeks earlier.

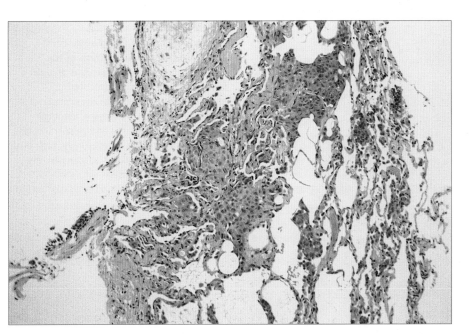

Figure 33.3
Higher power view of the peribronchial parenchyma shows the alveolar spaces filled with sheet-like collections of macrophages with minimal increase in alveolar wall thickness in the background.

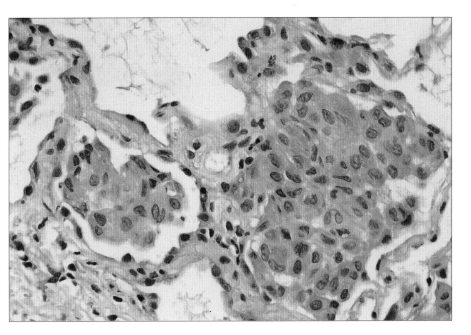

Figure 33.4
High-power view confirms these cells to be of macrophage appearance with faint brownish pigmentation of the cytoplasm and occasional admixed eosinophils. Parenchyma from another fragment of the same biopsy shows similar accumulated macrophages with mild thickening of the alveolar walls and type II pneumocyte hyperplasia. Subsequent transbronchial biopsies showed identical appearances.

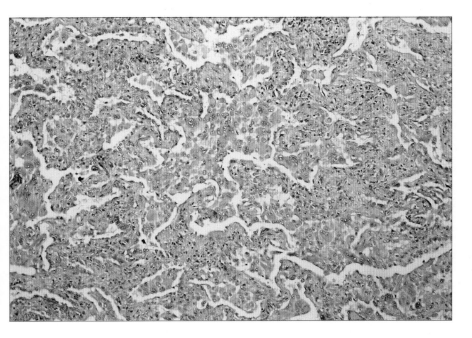

Figure 33.5
Both a preoperative diagnostic open lung biopsy and the lung explanted at single lung transplantation showed features of desquamative interstitial pneumonia (DIP) with some areas of typical usual interstitial pneumonia. The patient also had a history of asbestos exposure and scanty ferruginous bodies were present in both surgical specimens. The striking similarity of the DIP-like changes in the transbronchial biopsy (Figs 33.2–4) to the original pathology raise the possibility of recurrence. The role of the native lung with its asbestos load and the development of this contralateral pneumonitis remains speculative.

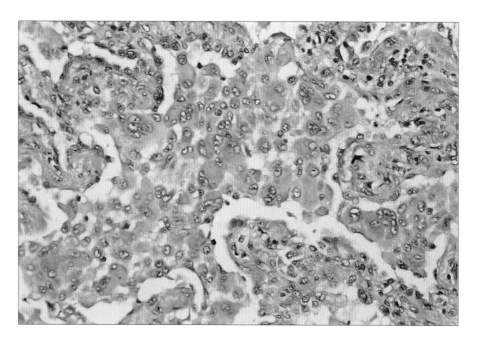

Figure 33.6
High-power view of the desquamative interstitial pneumonia reaction in the explanted lung with conspicuous alveolar filling by typical lightly pigmented macrophages and cuboidal hyperplasia of alveolar lining cells confirming identical appearances of the pre- and post-transplant pathologic processes. Interestingly, high-dose immunosuppression failed to dampen the recurrent DIP response.

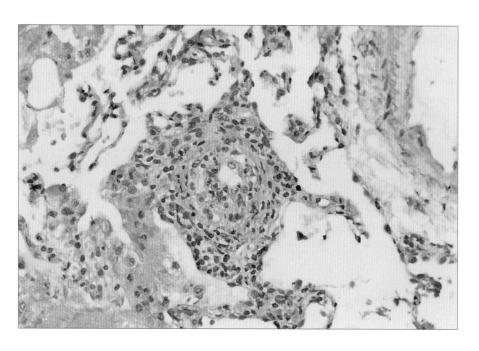

Figure 33.7
Transbronchial biopsy from a patient given a single lung transplant for emphysema. Several vessels in the biopsy showed infiltration of vessels involving full thickness of the vascular wall with splitting of the media by inflammatory cells and significant reduction in vascular lumen. No fibrinoid change was seen. The appearances are unlike acute rejection with perivascular cuffing and endothelialitis and do not show features of chronic vascular rejection with cellular infiltration admixed with fibrosis in the latter. The patient was found to have had systemic lupus erythematosis which has involved the grafted lung. This case emphasizes the need for full clinical history when interpreting transbronchial biopsies from the often complicated lung transplant patient.

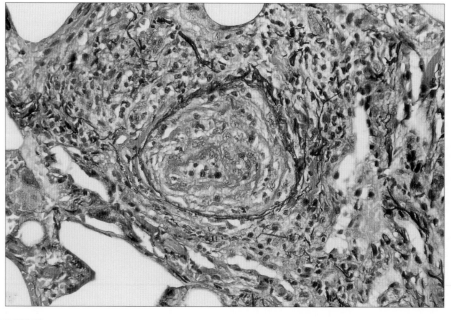

Figure 33.8
Elastic van Gieson-stained transbronchial biopsy showing involvement of grafted lung by systemic lupus erythematosis as in Fig. 33.7. Without the relevant clinical history the patient may have required open lung biopsy to elucidate the unusual transbronchial biopsy appearances.

FURTHER READING

Baz MA, Kussin PS, Van Trigt P, Davis RD, Roggli VL, Tapson VF. Recurrence of diffuse panbronchiolitis after lung transplantation. *Am J Respir Crit Care Med* 1995;**151**:895–8.

Bittman I, Dose TB, Müller C, Dienemann H, Vogelmeier C, Löhrs U. Lymphangiomatosis: Recurrence after single lung transplantation. *Hum Pathol* 1997;**26**:1420–23.

Brézillon S, Hamm H, Heilmann M *et al*. Decreased expression of the cystic fibrosis transmembrane conductance regulator protein in remodeled airway epithelium from lung transplanted patients. *Hum Pathol* 1997;**28**:944–52.

Gabbay E, Dark JH, Ashcroft T, Milne D, Gibson EGJ, Healy M, Corris PA. Recurrence of Langerhans' cell granulomatosis following lung transplantation. *Thorax* 1998;**53**:326–7.

Habib SB, Congleton J, Carr D *et al*. Recurrence of recipient Langerhans' cell histiocytosis following bilateral lung transplantation. *Thorax* 1998; **53**:323–5.

Hillerdal G, Nou E, Osterman K, Schmekel B. Sarcoidosis: epidemiology and prognosis. *Am Rev Respir Dis* 1984;**130**:29–30.

Johnson BA, Duncan SR, Ohori NO *et al*. Recurrence of sarcoidosis in pulmonary allograft recipients. *Am Rev Respir Dis* 1993;**148**:1373–7.

Judson MA. Lung transplantation for pulmonary sarcoidosis. *Eur Respir J* 1998;**11**:738–44.

Kalassian KG, Doyle R, Kao P, Ruoss S, Raffin TA. Pulmonary perspective. Lymphangioleiomyomatosis: New insights. *Am J Respir Crit Care Med* 1997;**155**:1183–86.

King MB, Jessurun J, Hertz MI. Recurrence of desquamative interstitial pneumonia after lung transplantation. *Am J Respir Crit Care Med* 1997;**156**:2003–5.

Kon OM, du Bois RM. Mycobacteria and sarcoidosis. *Thorax* 1996;**51**:530–3.

O'Brien JD, Lium JH, Parosa JG, Deyoung BR, Wick MR, Trulock EP. Lymphangiomatosis recurrence in the allograft after single-lung transplantation. *Am J Respir Crit Care Med* 1995;**151**:2033–36.

Padilla ML, Schilero GJ, Teirstein AS. Sarcoidosis and transplantation. *Sarcoidosis Vasc Diffuse Lung Dis* 1997;**14**:16–22.

Verleden GM, Sels F, Van Raemdonck D, Verbeken EK, Lerut T, Demedts M. Possible recurrence of desquamative interstitial pneumonitis in a single lung transplant recipient. *Eur Respir J* 1998;**11**:971–4.

Walker S, Mikhail G, Banner N *et al*. Medium Term Results of Lung Transplantation for End Stage Pulmonary Sarcoidosis. *Thorax* 1998;**53**:281–4.

Yeatman M, McNeil K, Smith JA *et al*. Lung transplantation in patients with systemic diseases: An eleven-year experience at Papworth Hospital. *J Heart Lung Transplant* 1996;**15**:144–9.

This process must be distinguished from obliterative bronchiolitis. It can exist as a purely intra-alveolar process or in the form of bronchiolitis obliterans organizing pneumonia (BOOP) in which both distal airways and parenchyma show intraluminal organizing granulation tissue polyps. Patients with a history of organizing pneumonia have an increased risk of obliterative bronchiolitis which may be related to common etiologies or risk factors or a genetic predisposition to fibrose after injury.

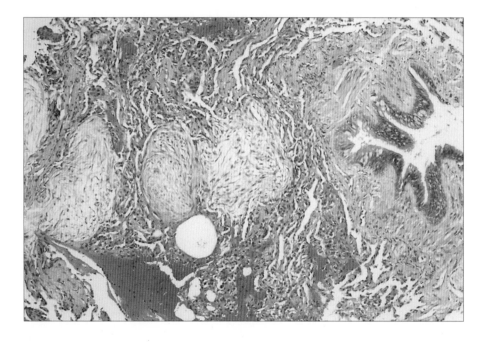

Figure 34.1
Transbronchial biopsy with several intra-alveolar fibroproliferative polyps of organizing pneumonia following infection. The process is clearly intraparenchymal without involvement of the adjacent airway.

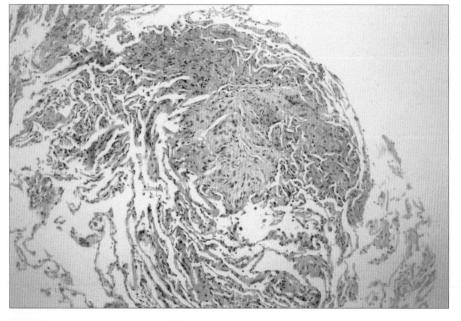

Figure 34.2
Transbronchial biopsy showing organizing pneumonia with loose fibrocellular tissue in intra-alveolar spaces. There is a history of infection which had incompletely resolved and a short course of steroids produced complete resolution. The information available from transbronchial biopsies allows appropriate use of steroids when enhanced immunosuppression for rejection is not required.

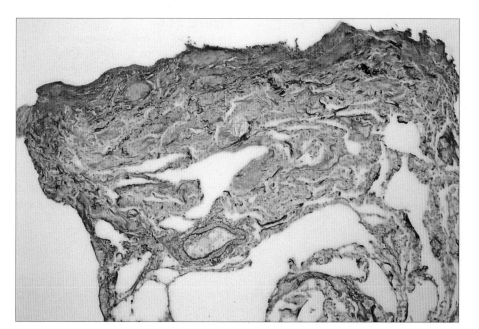

Figure 34.3
Low-power view of same lung fragment deeper into serial section showing intra-alveolar fibrosis of organizing pneumonia with pale staining collagen. Perls' elastic van Gieson stain.

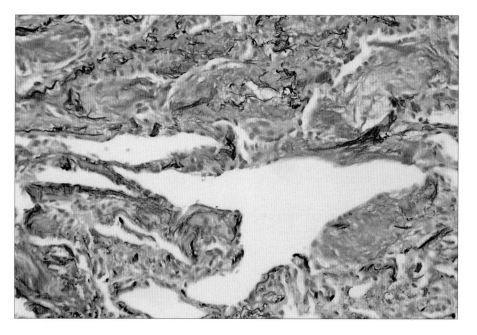

Figure 34.4
High-power view of intra-alveolar collagen of organizing pneumonia in a transbronchial biopsy. The collagen is fairly pale staining and there is no evidence of dense hyaline scarring. The patient recovered full lung function with further antibiotic treatment. Perls' elastic van Gieson stain.

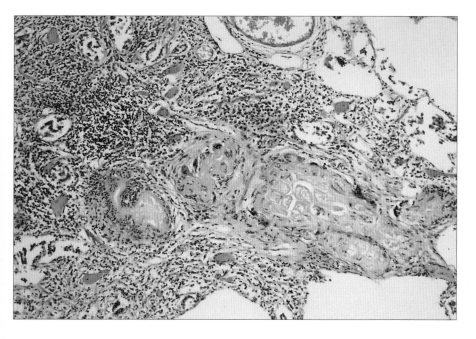

Figure 34.5
Organization of aspiration pneumonia with frequent foreign body type giant cells. This was such a persistent problem that surgical intervention was required but the aspiration only came to attention on this transbronchial biopsy for persistent cough and X-ray abnormalities.

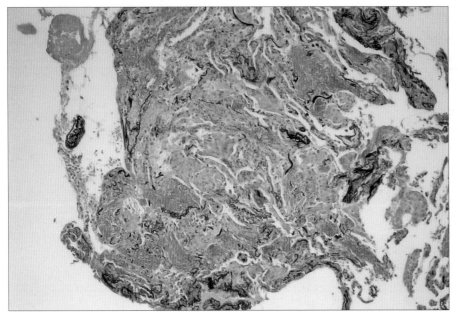

Figure 34.6
Intra-alveolar fibrosis following acute respiratory distress syndrome. These changes are often seen in several subsequent transbronchial biopsies after symptomatic improvement. Perls' elastic van Gieson stain

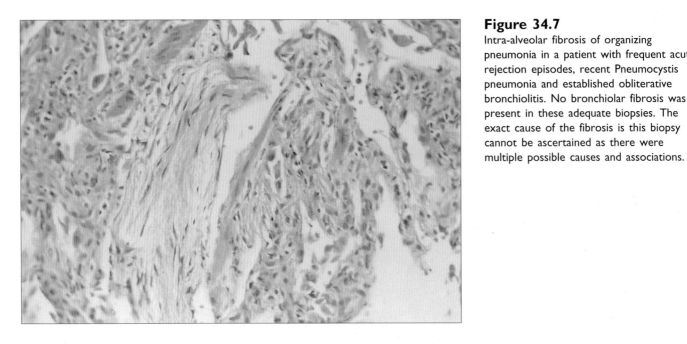

Figure 34.7
Intra-alveolar fibrosis of organizing pneumonia in a patient with frequent acute rejection episodes, recent Pneumocystis pneumonia and established obliterative bronchiolitis. No bronchiolar fibrosis was present in these adequate biopsies. The exact cause of the fibrosis is this biopsy cannot be ascertained as there were multiple possible causes and associations.

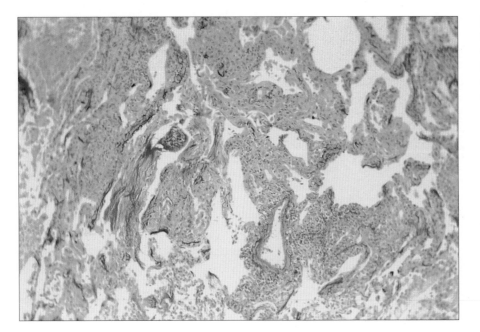

Figure 34.8
Same biopsies as Fig. 34.7, showing the value of a connective tissue stain is highlighting significant intra-alveolar fibrosis, clearly visible here at low-power. Perls' elastic van Gieson stain.

FURTHER READING

Abernathy EC, Hruban RH, Baumgartner WA, Reitz BA, Hutchins GM. The two forms of bronchiolitis obliterans in heart–lung transplant recipients. *Hum Pathol* 1991;**22**:1102–10.

Camus P, Lombard J-N, Perrichon M *et al*. Bronchiolitis obliterans organising pneumonia in patients taking acebutalol or amiodarone. *Thorax* 1989;**44**:711–15.

Chaparro C, Chamberlain D, Maurer J, Winton T, De Hoyos A, Kesten S. Bronchiolitis obliterans organising pneumonia (BOOP) in lung transplant patients. *Chest* 1996;**110**:1150–54.

Milne DS, Gascoigne AD, Ashcroft T *et al*. Organising pneumonia following pulmonary transplantation and the development of obliterative bronchiolitis. *Transplantation* 1994;**57**:1757–62.

Reid KR, McKenzie FN, Menkis AH *et al*. Importance of chronic aspiration in recipients of heart-lung transplants. *Lancet* 1990;**336**:206–8.

Siddiqui MT, Garrity ER, Husain AN. Bronchiolitis obliterans organising pneumonia-like reactions: A non-specific response or an atypical form of rejection or infection in lung allograft recipients. *Hum Pathol* 1996;**27**:714–19.

Yousem SA, Duncan S, Griffith B. Interstitial and airspace granulation tissue reaction in lung transplant recipients. *Am J Surg Path* 1992;**16**:877–84.

SECTION THIRTY-FIVE
NON-SPECIFIC HISTOLOGIC FEATURES

Transbronchial biopsies from lung transplant recipients often show non-specific histologic features. With improved postoperative management including new immunosuppressive regimes and the use of prophylactic antimicrobials, there is better control of previously common complications. As a result the proportion of transbronchial biopsies showing only non-specific features has increased and in some centers may represent the majority of biopsies. It is important not to overdiagnose non-specific features and to assess adequacy of the samples at all times. A non-specific transbronchial biopsy may be accompanied by a diagnostic bronchoalveolar lavage, microbiologic culture or serologic titer change, thereby allowing firm diagnosis for a particular clinical episode. There is also the very useful exclusion of other pathologies such as acute rejection and graft infection. In this way biopsies of non-specific histologic appearances may still be useful in the postoperative management of the patient. Assessment of these features is considerably easier for those pathologists familiar with general pulmonary pathology. As with all post-transplant transbronchial biopsies the usefulness is increased by good liaison with the clinicians and multidisciplinary discussion. Occasionally non-specific, non-diagnostic biopsies will need to be repeated if the clinical episode or deterioration remains unexplained and even less frequently may be an indication for an open biopsy in order to reach a firm diagnosis of unexplained clinical, functional or radiologic abnormalities.

Also included in this section are other unusual features on transbronchial biopsies which can be confusing for the unwary.

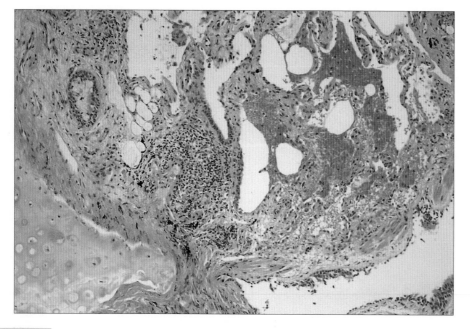

Figure 35.1

Transbronchial biopsy showing a common selection of non-specific features with intra-alveolar hemorrhage and macrophages. There is also a non-specific infiltrate of mononuclear cells beneath the bronchiolar epithelium and some anthracosis. The pinch artifact caused by the biopsy forceps is clearly seen and occasionally this can obscure a diagnostic area in the biopsy. Also present are the round spaces known as 'bubble artefact' which are common in transbronchial biopsies and should not be confused with deposits of lipid.

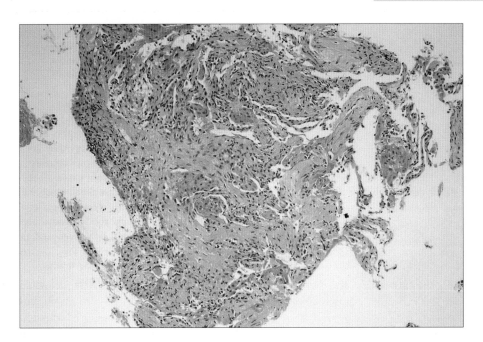

Figure 35.2
Another transbronchial biopsy showing intra-alveolar fibrin and macrophages. The biopsy also shows collapse. There is no definite intra-alveolar fibrosis of organizing pneumonia but there is interstitial widening of alveolar walls. This appearance could be in keeping with recent infection, but no organisms were seen or cultured and the patient improved without specific treatment.

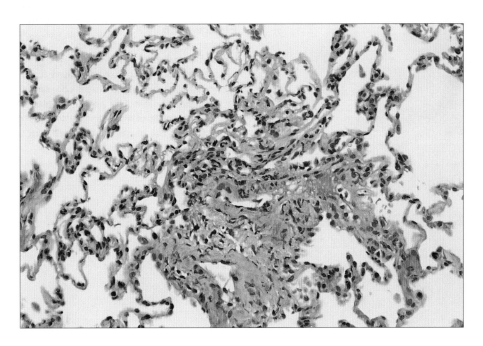

Figure 35.3
High-power of transbronchial biopsy showing an area of interstitial infiltration by mononuclear cells and occasional polymorphs which does not amount to perivascular cuffing. There is mild type II cell hyperplasia in all the alveoli. No cause is identified for these changes and no helpful features to direct treatment.

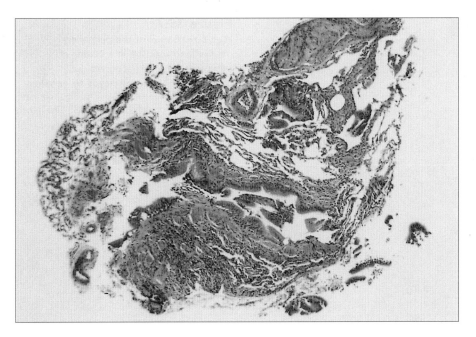

Figure 35.4
A low-power view of a transbronchial biopsy from a patient with decreased pulmonary function. There is a non-specific infiltrate around the central bronchiole with extension into parenchyma which shows collapse and fibrosis. There is no evidence of acute rejection, opportunistic infection nor of airways infection on microbiological culture. The most likely cause of symptoms in association with these non-specific findings is airways infection and empirical treatment with antibiotics produced clinical improvements.

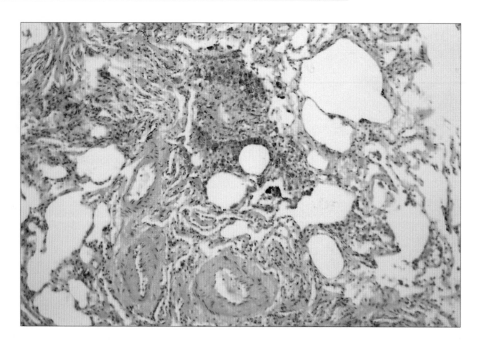

Figure 35.5
Another common non-specific finding is the presence of hemosiderin laden alveolar macrophages which may be related to previous episodes of inflammation, hemorrhage or even previous biopsies. In combined heart–lung grafts it is also possible that these could on occasion be due to heart failure. In this biopsy they are associated with a non-specific mononuclear cell infiltrate which is not perivascular. The arteriolar vessels are thick-walled, which is another common but entirely non-specific finding. This latter change should always be interpreted cautiously and only diagnosed as chronic vascular rejection when the appropriate transmural, including intimal, changes are present with fibrosis.

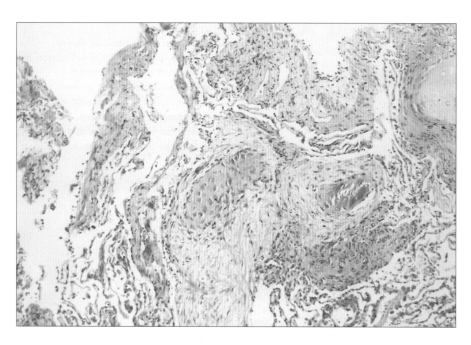

Figure 35.6
Another feature seen in transbronchial biopsies occasionally is the formation of metaplastic bone. This may be related to previous pulmonary hemorrhage, congestion or thromboembolism. It is not uncommon but appears to be of little clinical significance. It can be seen in patients with repeated biopsies showing extensive organizing pneumonia.

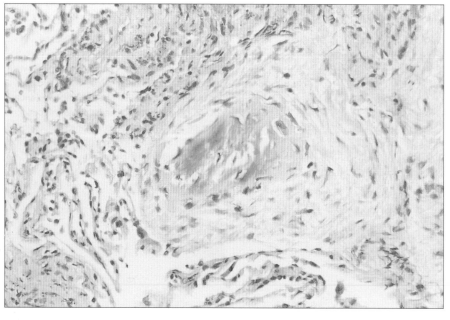

Figure 35.7
High-power view of the pulmonary ossification occurring in a setting of otherwise minimally abnormal lung parenchyma. No action needs to be taken.

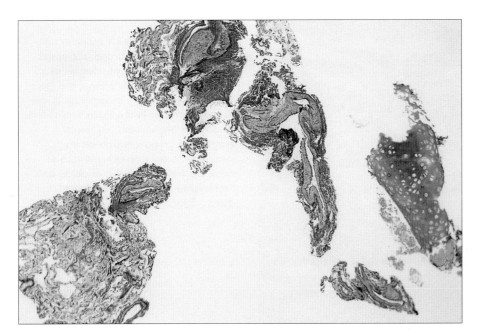

Figure 35.8
Transbronchial biopsy showing another cause of hemorrhage. Several of the biopsy fragments consist of arterial wall and the procedure had to be curtailed due to brisk hemorrhage. This is a recognized complication of transbronchial biopsy and it is helpful to report to the bronchoscopist as soon as possible the presence of significant vessel wall. Perls' elastic van Gieson stain.

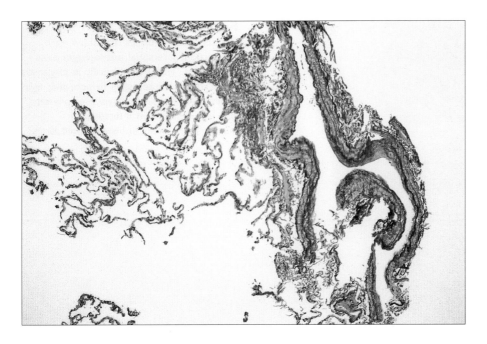

Figure 35.9
High-power view of Perls' elastic van Gieson stain showing the biopsied vessel together with some unremarkable attached parenchyma.

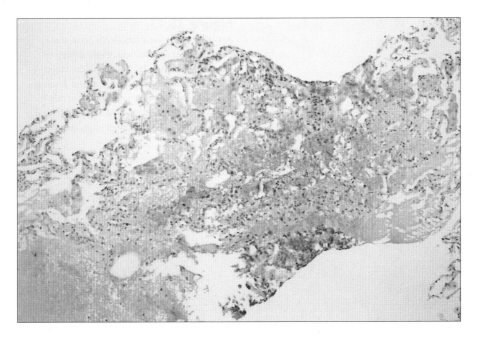

Figure 35.10
A fragment of transbronchial parenchyma in the same biopsy series shows parenchymal hemorrhage due to the damaged vessel. In some cases a specific diagnosis will also be present. In this situation of artefactual hemorrhage, the biopsy may need to be read with an inadequate number of fragments and it may be necessary to recommend re-biopsy if only non-specific features are present.

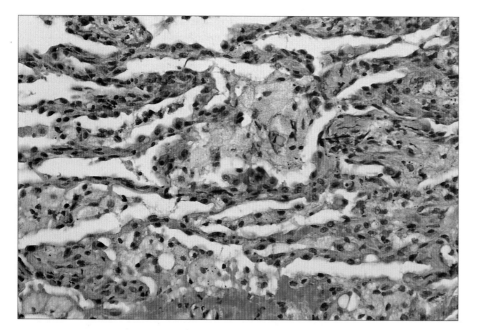

Figure 35.11
Foamy macrophages are a common non-specific finding in transbronchial biopsies. They generally indicate obstruction of a small airway and should prompt a diligent search for obliterative bronchiolitis in the biopsy fragments. In the absence of definite obliterative bronchiolitis but clinical evidence of bronchiolitis obliterans syndrome, foamy macrophages such as these are highly suggestive of obliterative bronchiolitis as the cause of clinical deterioration.

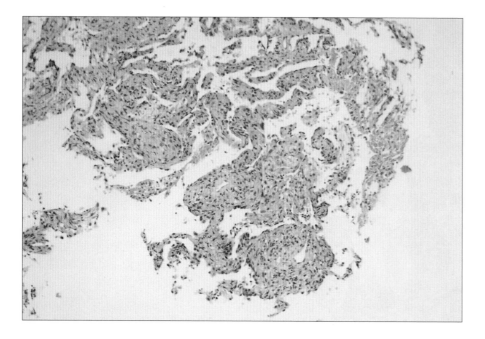

Figure 35.12
Transbronchial biopsies may show conspicuous interstitial macrophages as in this patient. This is non-specific in diagnostic terms, but it is interesting to note that this patient with alpha-1-antitrypsin emphysema also had conspicuous interstitial macrophages focally in his explanted lungs.

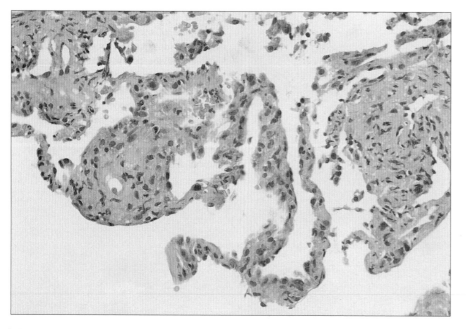

Figure 35.13
A high-power view confirms that the macrophages are almost exclusively interstitial with a faintly granulomatous appearance. This is a non-specific finding which should always prompt a search for organisms particularly of a mycobacterial nature. None was seen or cultured from this case.

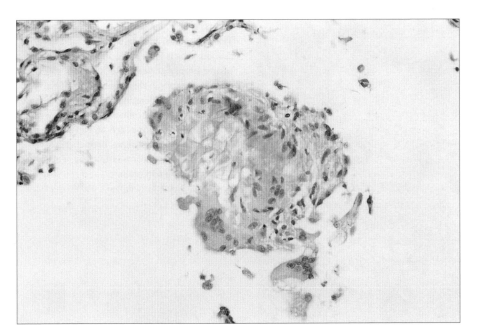

Figure 35.14
Macrophages in transbronchial biopsies in lung recipients may form granulomas such as this foreign body giant cell granuloma which contains pigmented material of uncertain nature. This non-specific finding raises the possibility of aspiration which is important to report to the clinician. Aspiration is an under-recognized, but important complication in lung transplant recipients.

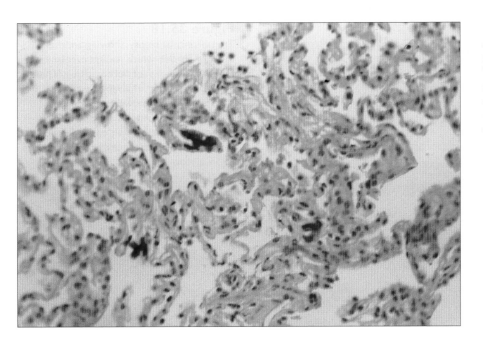

Figure 35.15
A transbronchial biopsy showing three megakaryocytes within pulmonary capillaries. This is not uncommon in transplant recipients. They should not cause diagnostic difficulty if correctly recognized, but in our referral practice have been confused with viral inclusions and cytopathic effects.

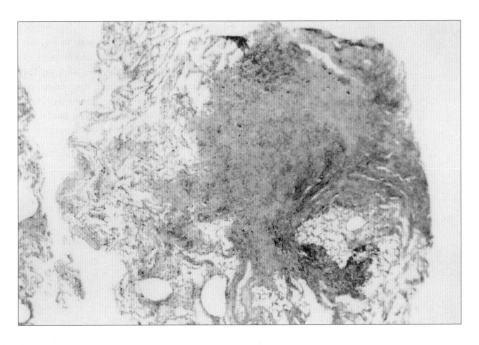

Figure 35.16
The assessment of fibrosis in transbronchial biopsies is fraught with difficulty, but various types can be recognized. This low-power view shows nodular fibrosis in a patient with many previous episodes of acute rejection, cytomegalovirus pneumonitis and deterioration in lung function. This nodule of parenchymal fibrosis should not be confused with obliterative bronchiolitis. This biopsy also shows a focus of persistent A2 acute rejection.

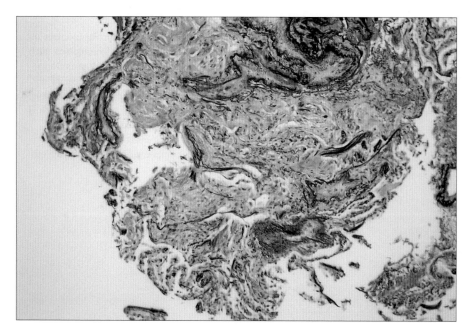

Figure 35.17

Transbronchial biopsy showing intra-alveolar fibrosis which is present in a single fragment of the biopsy series only but fulfils the criteria for organizing pneumonia. This diagnostic label does not however give any clues as to specific etiology. Patients with organizing pneumonia are at increased risk of developing obliterative bronchiolitis though the mechanism is unclear. Perls' elastic van Gieson stain.

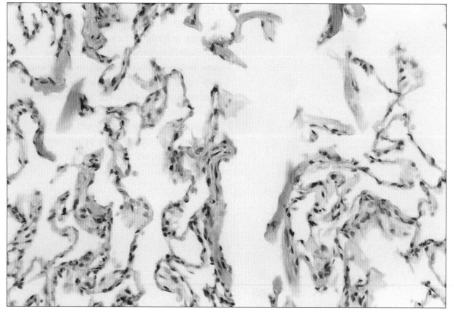

Figure 35.18

Transbronchial biopsy showing another form of fibrosis which is intraalveolar in the form of 'cushions' of fibrous tissue. There is fibrotic thickening of alveolar walls also. This patient was known to suffer from obliterative bronchiolitis and this pattern would be consistent with circumferential narrowing of a respiratory bronchiole close to an alveolar duct.

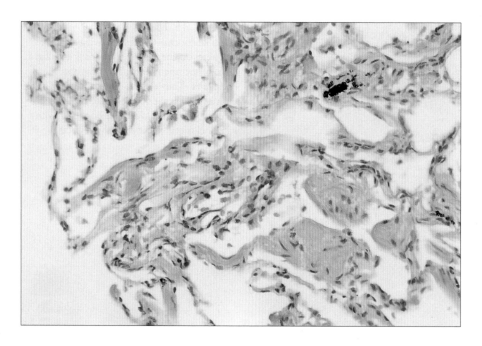

Figure 35.19

The alveolar wall fibrosis as seen in Fig. 35.18 is entirely non-specific and is seen even in clinically stable patients with no loss of function. The transplanted lung does not appear to develop a diffuse interstitial fibrosis of fibrosing alveolitis type in response to injury.

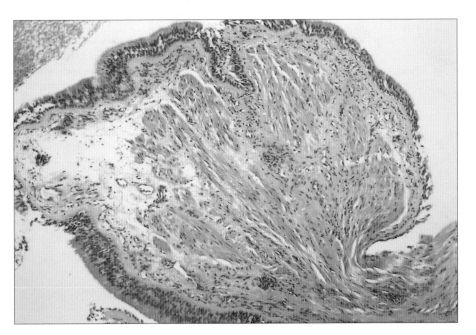

Figure 35.20
Transbronchial biopsy showing non-specific features in the mucosal fragment of smooth muscle hyperplasia, a mild subepithelial inflammatory infiltrate and prominent eosinophilic basement membrane thickening. These features are sometimes associated with reversible airflow obstruction mimicking asthma and can be seen in patients with chronic *Pseudomonas* or *Aspergillus* infection. Stable asymptomatic recipients may also show these features.

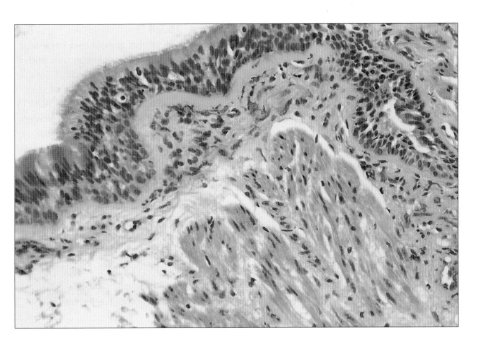

Figure 35.21
High-power view of the bronchial changes in Fig. 35.20 showing smooth muscle hyperplasia, inflammation and basement membrane thickening. Occasional inflammatory cells are present in the epithelium which retains its normal ciliated surface.

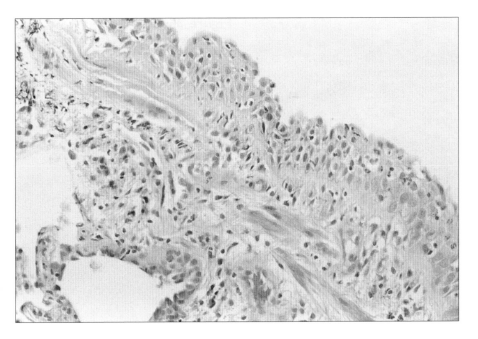

Figure 35.22
Squamous metaplasia of the surface respiratory epithelium is very common in lung transplant recipients. It may be infiltrated by polymorphs as in this case which generally indicates airways infection. The high prevalence of squamous metaplasia in these patients with decreased mucociliary clearance as a result may contribute to the high incidence of bacterial infections.

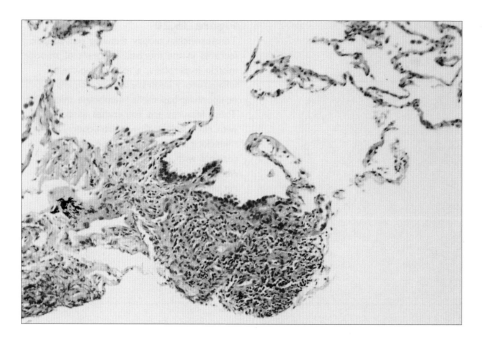

Figure 35.23
A transbronchial biopsy at low-power showing a structured area of lymphoid tissue in which vessels can be seen which is subepithelial and apparently bronchiolar in distribution.

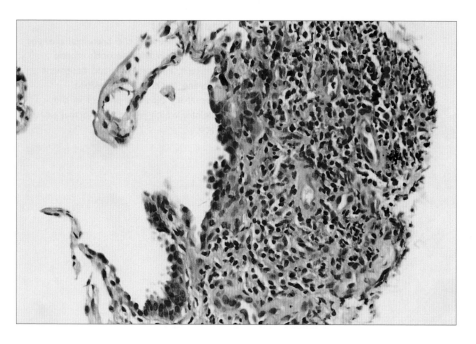

Figure 35.24
Higher power of this area shows organized lymphoid tissue with frequent vessels and occasional anthracotic pigmented macrophages. This is a small focus of bronchus-associated lymphoid tissue (BALT) which should not be confused with airways rejection. Its presence is a non-specific finding but it has been shown to be depleted in chronic lung rejection in some studies.

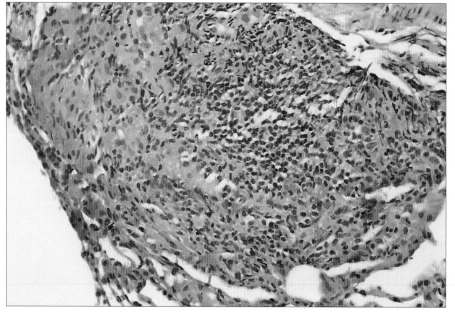

Figure 35.25
High-power view of BALT in another case. The association of organized lymphoid tissue with prominent vessels and pigmented macrophages should enable the differential diagnosis to be made from other causes of mononuclear cells in airways, particularly infections and acute rejection.

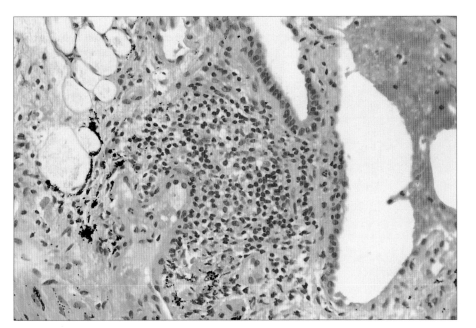

Figure 35.26
A high-power view of the case shown in Fig. 35.1 showing that this lymphoid collection is also associated with vessels one of which shows endothelialitis. The anthracotic pigment is also a helpful feature in determining that this is most likely to be BALT in origin. In larger airways the vessels that are part of the normal airway structure should not be misinterpreted as part of a BALT lesion.

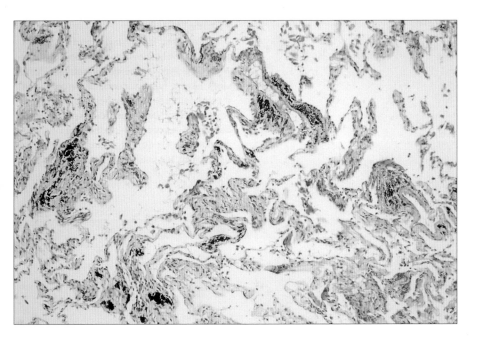

Figure 35.27
Low-power view of a transbronchial biopsy from a patient who received a donor lung from a smoker. Several deposits of anthracotic and smoker's-type pigment are seen consistent with respiratory bronchiolitis.

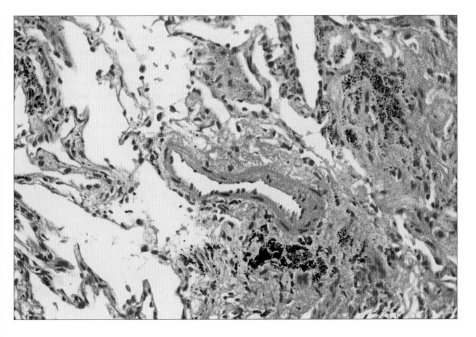

Figure 35.28
A higher power view shows the pigment in greater detail some of which is perivascular and the remainder peribronchiolar. There is a mixture of brownish smoker's pigment and carbon. This lesion seems to be of little clinical significance in the graft. It is seen more commonly as smoker donors are used more frequently than previously when there was a larger donor pool and fewer potential recipients.

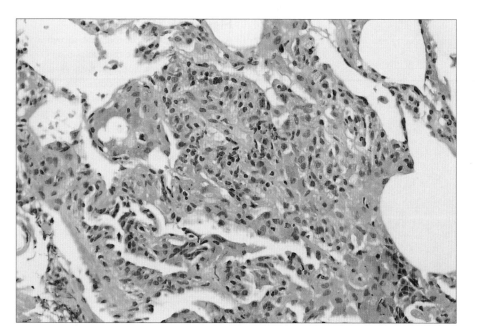

Figure 35.29

A transbronchial biopsy taken at 2 weeks showing pigmented macrophage accumulation with polymorphs, lymphocytes and occasional eosinophils, the mononuclear cell infiltrate appearing to be centered on a vessel. The donor was a child who had smoked, but the graft was not expected to show respiratory bronchiolitis of this degree. The possibility of concomitant acute rejection has to be considered, but it cannot be graded in the presence of these other pathologic changes. The biopsy did not show typical perivascular infiltrates of acute rejection elsewhere. The patient grew bacteria from the airway and made a complete response to antibiotic therapy alone.

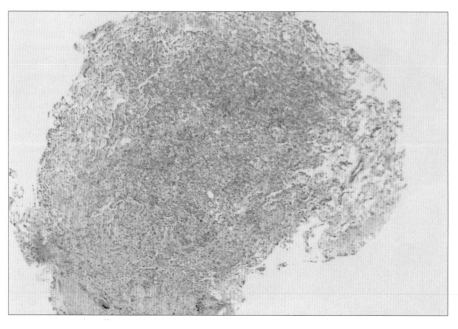

Figure 35.30

Transbronchial biopsy taken at 10 days postoperatively showing organizing thrombi which are likely to be donor-related. Donor lungs have a high incidence of thrombi and thromboemboli despite their generally young age and previous healthy state. Small peripheral lesions such as the one illustrated here do not seem to have clinical significance for the transplanted lungs.

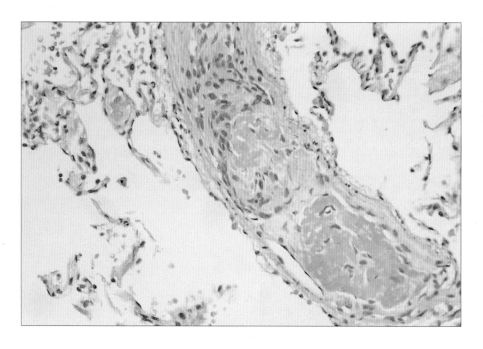

Figure 35.31

Another fragment of the same biopsy series shows obvious consolidation at low-power as explanation for the clinical deterioration and radiographic opacification. The consolidation appears diffuse with no perivascular predilection.

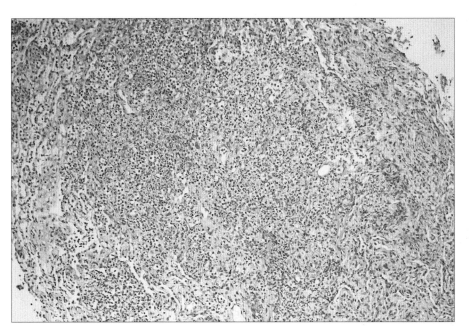

Figure 35.32
Higher power confirms a florid acute pneumonia which is very likely to have been donor transmitted. Suitable but unused donor lungs frequently show acute purulent bronchitis and bronchiolitis which is to be expected in view of the sequelae of brain death and assisted ventilation. This patient presented with a clinical and radiographic picture which would have been entirely consistent with acute pulmonary rejection and therefore emphasizes the importance of biopsy to establish the correct diagnosis. An incorrect clinical diagnosis would have led to enhanced immunosuppression in the face of severe infection.

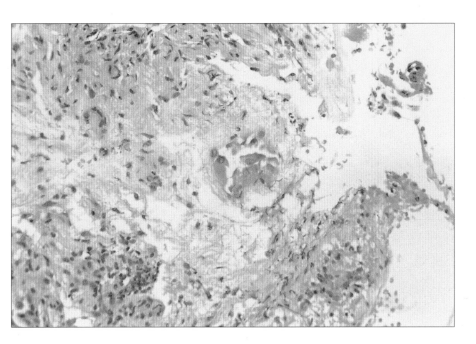

Figure 35.33
Transbronchial biopsies may include mesothelium from the pleura (center of field) which should be correctly identified and reported to the bronchoscopist because of the risk of pneumothorax. Reactive mesothelium in the first few weeks after transplantation can cause considerable confusion (as indeed is the case when reactive mesothelium from the pericardium is included in endomyocardial biopsies).

Box 30 Transbronchial lung biopsy

Common artefacts
- Atelectasis – delayed fixation
  – confuses diagnosis
- Intra-alveolar hemorrhage
- Bubble artefact
- Pleural samples included

Box 31 Transbronchial lung biopsy

Non-specific findings
- DAD – full spectrum of changes not seen on small biopsies
- Hyaline membranes often absent
- Interstitial pneumonia
- Fibrosis
- Acute and chronic inflammation
- Hemorrhage/hemosiderin

FURTHER READING

Bernardi P, Delsedime L. Bellis D, Mollo F. Atypical changes of respiratory epithelium after heart-lung transplantation. *Path Res Pract* 1989;**184**:514–18.

Gould SJ, Isaacson PG. Bronchus-associated lymphoid tissue (BALT) in human fetal and infant lung. *J Pathol* 1993;**169**:229–34.

Hruban RH, Beschorner WE, Baumgartner WA *et al.* Depletion of bronchus-associated lymphoid tissue with lung allograft rejection. *Am J Pathol* 1988;**132**:6.

Lee AGL, Wagner FM, Chen M-F, Serrick C, Giaid A, Shennib H. A novel charcoal-induced model of obliterative bronchiolitis-like lesions: implications of chronic non-specific airway inflammation in the development of posttransplantation obliterative bronchiolitis. *J Thorac Cardiovasc Surg* 1998;**115**:522–7.

Marques LJ, Teschler H, Guzman J, Costabel U. Smoker's lung transplanted to a non-smoker. *Am J Respir Crit Care Med* 1997;**156**:1700–2.

Nishio JN, Lynch JP. Fiberoptic bronchoscopy in the immunocompromised host: the significance of a 'nonspecific' transbronchial biopsy. *Am Rev Respir Dis* 1980;**121**:307–12

Pfitzmann R, Hummel M, Grauhan O *et al.* Acute graft-versus-host disease after human heart-lung transplantation: a case report. *J Thorac Cardiovasc Surg* 1997;**114**:285–7.

Stewart S, Ciulli F, Wells F, Wallwork J. Pathology of unused donor lungs. *Transplant Proc* 1993;**25**:1167–1168.

BRONCHOALVEOLAR LAVAGE CYTOLOGY

Bronchoalveolar lavage (BAL) is a non-invasive technique which has been applied both to experimental and clinical lung transplantation. It can be used to assess the inflammatory and immune responses of the transplanted lung. Most studies of bronchoalveolar lavage assume that the cells obtained are representative of those within the lung parenchyma and in lung transplantation this has been confirmed by studies looking at biopsies and synchronous lavages. In the clinical diagnostic setting bronchoalveolar lavage has a major role in the diagnosis of opportunistic infection involving both cytologic examination and culture. Diagnosis by cytologic examination of the fluid can be rapid. Care must be taken however not to over interpret the presence of potential colonizers such as *Candida*, *Aspergillus* and cytomegalovirus (CMV). The lavage should be reported together with the accompanying biopsy in order to determine the significance of any opportunistic organisms seen. The proliferation of more sensitive techniques including immunohistochemistry, *in situ* DNA hybridization and polymerase chain reaction for diagnosis may not be helpful in making the distinction between colonization, incidental infection and a true pneumonitis. The accompanying inflammatory cells in the lavage may be helpful in assessing the significance of any organism. CMV inclusion-containing cells in an inflammatory lavage may be more significant than those with a near normal cell count.

In our experience routine H & E staining of the bronchoalveolar lavage or bronchial aspirate with a routine Grocott stain of all fluids has allowed a satisfactory yield of diagnoses. Viral inclusions such as CMV and HSV are easily identified in H & E stained material and the Grocott stain is useful for *Aspergillus*, *Candida* and *Pneumocystis*. The use of H & E cytology simplifies the identification of eosinophils in lavage fluid and Charcot–Leyden crystals.

The commonest findings at lavage cytology in the transplant population are non-specific and non-diagnostic. The cellular profile is always abnormal compared with non-transplanted controls in that the cellularity overall is increased and there is an excess of alveolar macrophages. Purulent aspirates are very common particularly where a true wedged alveolar lavage has not been carried out and larger airways have been sampled.

In the early days of lung transplantation the cell populations were analysed with functional testing of lymphocytes performed on lavage samples. Most of the donor lymphocytes in the graft seem to be replaced by recipient cells in the first 6 weeks, although donor cells may persist for as long as 32 weeks. Acute rejection occurs with lower incidence after the period when donor lymphocytes are easily found in the graft. During acute rejection episodes, lymphocytes obtained by bronchoalveolar lavage are cytolytic to donor spleen cells showing spontaneous proliferation and interleukin 2 responsiveness. However these features are also seen during episodes of infection and neither absolute count, cellular profiles or cytolytic function can distinguish infection from rejection reliably. High lymphocyte counts greater than 15% are supportive of a diagnosis of rejection but are found in less than 25% of rejection episodes. Also neutrophils are increased in both rejection and infection. Lymphocyte phenotype studies have shown that CD3 and CD8 cells are increased in both acute and chronic rejection, but with considerable overlap between rejecting and infected grafts. CD8 cells always predominate but this may be because they are the most common cells in both normal and diseased respiratory epithelium. BAL cells cultured from patients undergoing acute rejection show a predominance of CD4 phenotypes with class 2 directed reactivity which contrasts with a CD8 prominence with class 1 directed reactivity in patients with obliterative bronchiolitis. The high rate of common and opportunistic infection in lung transplant recipients and the immune modulatory effects of viral pathogens such as CMV are likely to confound attempts to realize the full potential of lavage studies in the diagnosis of rejection and other graft complications.

Recently the neutrophil has been studied in BAL, particularly indices of activation and is being shown to be important in the pathogenesis of obliterative bronchiolitis.

Other forms of cytologic diagnosis such as fine needle aspiration cytology can be applied to the investigation of new nodules following lung transplantation. The findings are very similar to those in other immunocompromised hosts, but the higher likelihood of post-transplant lymphoproliferative disorder should be remembered in the differential diagnosis.

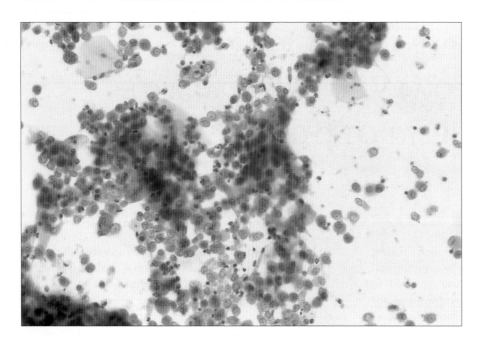

Figure 36.1

A typical postoperative lavage from a lung transplant recipient stained with H & E. The predominant cell is a macrophage with many containing hemosiderin pigment. Normal bronchial epithelial cells can be identified together with occasional red cells and lymphocytes. Very occasional oral squamous cells are also present. Formal counting of cells to construct profiles requires strict bronchoalveolar lavage rather than the commoner bronchial aspiration.

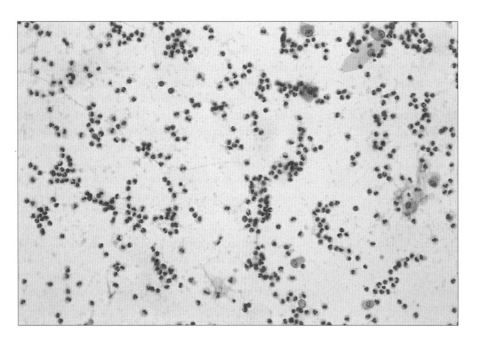

Figure 36.2

Bronchial aspirate from a lung transplant recipient with pyrexia and diminished lung function. There are pigmented macrophages, but the predominant abnormality is an excess of polymorphs. *Staphylococcus* was grown from sample and the patient made a recovery on antibiotic therapy. The high cellularity of the aspirate can be appreciated even at low-power. The implications of activated neutrophils for survival of the grafts are new areas for research.

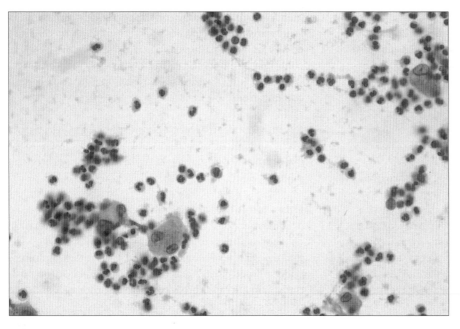

Figure 36.3

Higher power of the same aspirate confirms that the predominant cell is the polymorph. The finding of such a purulent aspirate can be very helpful when interpreting the paired transbronchial biopsy which showed polymorphs within the airway epithelium and infrequent scattered polymorphs in the parenchyma.

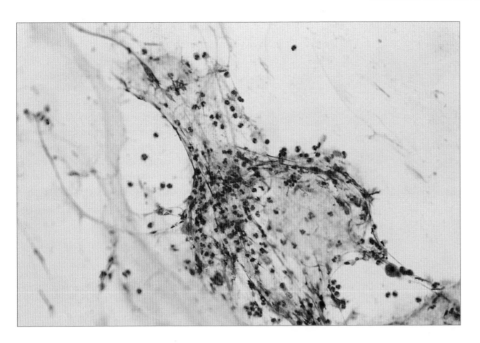

Figure 36.4
The lavage is often mucoid as well as inflammatory. This aspirate contains numerous polymorphs but also some eosinophils and a poorly defined Charcot–Leyden crystal.

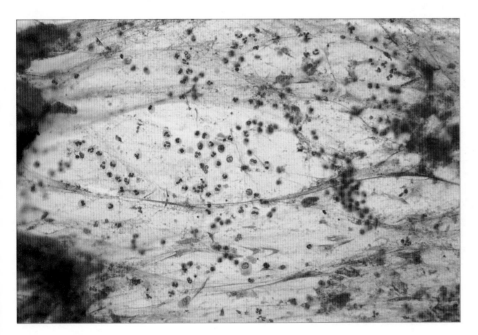

Figure 36.5
Another area from the same lavage preparation shows polymorphs with occasional eosinophils and much granular necrotic debris in the background. Charcot–Leyden crystals shown as elongated eosinophilic needle-like structures are very easily seen. Although no fungus was seen in this specimen in the paired silver stained slide *Aspergillus fumigatus* was cultured 2 days later. Symptoms improved with antifungal treatment and inhaled steroids.

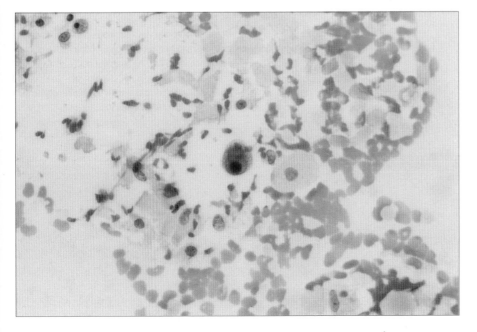

Figure 36.6
Hemorrhagic aspirate showing a CMV inclusion in an alveolar macrophage. Few inflammatory cells accompany the virally infected cell. The hemorrhage is suggestive of a pneumonitis, but can also be seen commonly as a result of bronchoscopic trauma. In this case the significance of the CMV infection was determined by a florid diffuse CMV alveolitis in the paired biopsy. In the absence of that biopsy a confident diagnosis of CMV pneumonitis could not be made on the lavage alone.

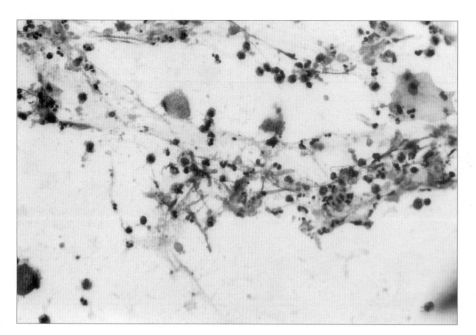

Figure 36.7
An inflammatory aspirate with polymorphs, macrophages and debris. In the center of the field faintly hematoxyphilic hyphae of *Aspergillus* can just be made out. The H & E staining allows *Aspergillus* to be identified in some cases with the mandatory Grocott stain ensuring accurate diagnosis and identification of the fungus. Very small amounts of fungal hyphae particularly if fragmented can be overlooked if Grocott staining is not performed in every case.

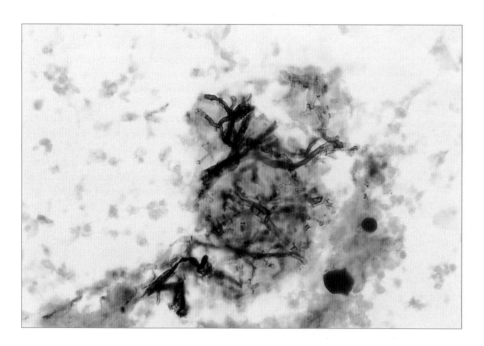

Figure 36.8
Grocott silver stain of *Aspergillus* allows the diagnostic features to be identified, namely dichotomous branching and septate, broad and regular hyphae. It is always advisable to correlate with microbiological findings which will allow an assessment of fungal load through the number of colony forming units.

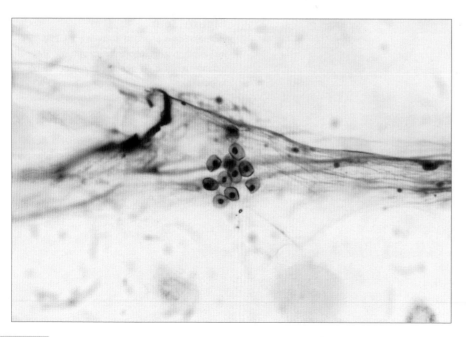

Figure 36.9
Bronchoalveolar lavage from a patient with granulomatous *Pneumocystis carinii* pneumonia following augmented immunosuppression. A cluster of pneumocysts is present. It is more common in lung transplant recipients to see infrequent scattered single pneumocysts.

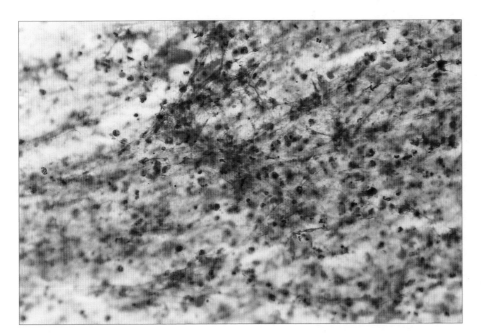

Figure 36.10
Extremely necrotic and purulent aspirate is strongly suggestive of infection, particularly by Herpes simplex or more unusually *Aspergillus*. Appearances such as these should prompt a search for viral inclusions and be correlated with virologic studies.

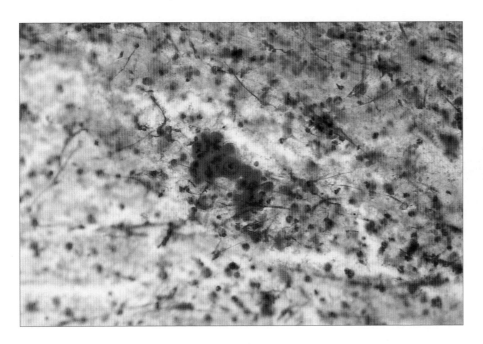

Figure 36.11
The necrotic debris in the aspirate includes a cluster of virally-infected epithelial cells, consistent with herpes simplex virus which was confirmed by immunofluorescence and culture.

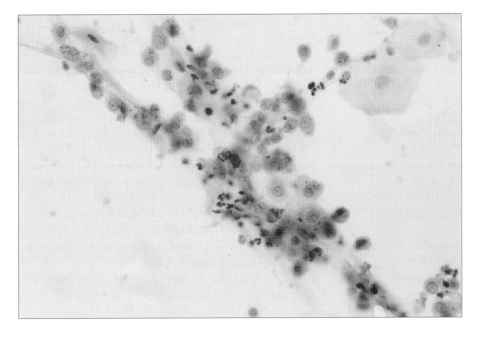

Figure 36.12
A lavage from a different patient showing diagnostic inclusions (intranuclear) of herpes simplex virus in epithelial cells. Rarely in the respiratory tract, infected cells will be multinucleated.

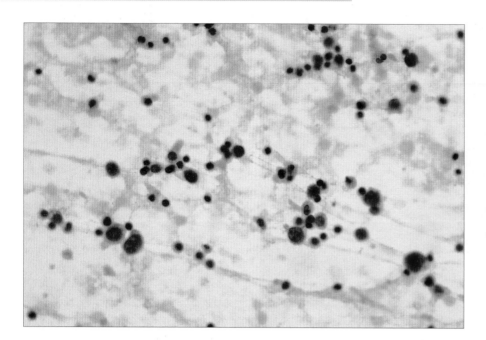

Figure 36.13
An H & E stained pleural fluid from a patient with a new radiographic mass in his transplanted lung. This was shown at bronchoscopy and later at open biopsy to be post-transplant lymphoproliferative disease. The pleural effusion is clearly due to involvement of the pleural space by a similar tumour. Highly atypical enlarged lymphoid cells are readily recognized. Malignancy is a rare cause of pleural effusions often lung transplantation. Effusions are common in episodes of acute rejection but are generally not sampled and clear with immunosuppression.

FURTHER READING

Chamberlain DW, Braude AC, Rebuck AS. A critical evaluation of bronchoalveolar lavage: criteria for identifying unsatisfactory specimens. *Acta Cytol* 1987;**31**:599–605.

Clelland CA, Higenbottam TW, Monk JA, Scott JP, Smyth RL, Wallwork J. Bronchoalveolar lavage lymphocytes in relation to transbronchial biopsy in heart-lung transplants. *Transplant Proc* 1990;**22**:1479.

Clelland CA, Higenbottam TW, Stewart S *et al.* Bronchoalveolar lavage and transbronchial lung biopsy during acute rejection and infection in heart–lung transplant patients. *Am Rev Respir Dis* 1993;**147**:1386–92.

Crim C, Keller CA, Dunphy CH, Maluf HM, Ohar JA. Flow cytometric analysis of lung lymphocytes in lung transplant recipient. *Am J Respir Crit Care Med* 1996;**153**:1041–6.

Davey DD, Gulley ML, Walker WP, Zaleski S. Cytologic findings in posttransplant lymphoproliferative disease. *Acta Cytol* 1990;**34**:304–10.

Delvenne P, Arrese JE, Thiry A, Borlée-Hermans G, Piérard GE, Boniver J. Detection of Cytomegalovirus, *Pneumocystis carinii*, and *Aspergillus* species in bronchoalveolar lavage fluid. *Am J Clin Pathol* 1993;**100**:414–18.

Holland VA, Cagle PT, Windsor NT, Noon GP, Greenberg SD, Lawrence EC. Lymphocyte subset populations in bronchiolitis obliterans after heart-lung transplantation. *Transplantation* 1990;**50**:955–9.

Judson MA, Handy JR, Sahn SA. Pleural Effusion from Acute Lung Rejection. *Chest* 1997;**111**:1128–30.

Judson MA, Sahn SA. The pleural space and the organ transplantation. *Am J Respir Crit Care Med* 1996;**153**:1153–65.

Martin WF, Smith TF, Bruntinel WM, Cockerill FR, Douglas WM. Role of bronchoalveolar lavage in the assessment of opportunistic pulmonary infections: Utility and complications. *Mayo Clinic Proc* 1987;**62**:549–57.

Maurer JR, Gough E, Chamberlain DW, Patterson GA, Grossman RF. Sequential bronchoalveolar lavage studies from patients undergoing double lung and heart-lung transplant. *Transplant Proc* 1989;**21**:2585–7.

Paradis IL, Grgurich WF, Dummer JS, Dekker A, Dauber JH. Rapid detection of cytomegalovirus pneumonia from lung lavage cells. *Am Rev Respir Dis* 1988;**138**:697–702.

Paradis IL, Marrari M, Zeevi A, Duquesnoy RJ, Griffith BP, Hardesty RL, Dauber JH. HLA phenotype of lung lavage cells following heart-lung transplantation. *Heart Transplant* 1985;**4**:422–5.

Rabinowich H, Zeevi A, Yousem SA *et al.* Alloreactivity of lung biopsy and bronchoalveolar lavage-derived lymphocytes from pulmonary transplant patients: Correlation with acute rejection and bronchiolitis obliterans. *Clin Transplant* 1990;**4**:376–84.

Reinsmoen NL, Bolman RM, Savik K, Butters K, Hertz M. Differentiation of Class I and Class II-directed donor-specific alloreactivity in bronchoalveolar lavage lymphocytes from lung transplant recipients. *Transplantation* 1992;**53**:181–9.

Riise GC, Andersson BA, Kjellström C *et al.* Persistent high BAL fluid granulocyte activation marker levels as early indicators of bronchiolitis obliterans after lung transplant. *Eur Respir J* 1999;**14**:1123–30.

Uberti-Foppa C, Lillo F, Terreni MR *et al.* Cytomegalovirus pneumonia in AIDS patients. Value of cytomegalovirus culture from BAL fluid and correlation with lung disease. *Chest* 1998;**113**:919–23.

Walts AE, Marchevski AM, Morgan M. Pulmonary cytology in lung: recent trends in laboratory utilization. *Diagn Cytopathol* 1991;**7**:353–8.

Winter JB, Clelland C, Gouw ASH, Prop J. Distinct phenotypes of infiltrating cells during acute and chronic lung rejection in human heart–lung transplant. *Transplantation* 1995;**59**:63–9.

Zeevi A, Fung JJ, Paradis IL *et al.* Lymphocytes of bronchoalveolar lavages from heart–lung transplant recipients. *Heart Transplant* 1985;**4**:417–21.

SECTION THIRTY-SEVEN

OPEN LUNG BIOPSIES

Bronchoscopy is the most widely used and accepted method for the investigation of complications of lung transplantation. Transbronchial biopsy and bronchoalveolar lavage detect rejection and/or infection with a high specificity and sensitivity. Transbronchial biopsies should always be interpreted in the light of clinical, radiologic and microbiologic findings in view of the wide differential diagnosis and lack of specificity of some of the histopathologic features such as perivascular infiltrates. Many studies have looked at the yield of bronchoscopic diagnosis in clinically-directed versus surveillance or protocol biopsies. Generally speaking the higher grades of acute rejection are seen in symptomatic patients, although it is not uncommon to see acute rejection above the treatment threshold in protocol biopsies. Some patients undergoing protocol biopsies do however have symptoms and signs when clinically assessed at the time of their procedure and therefore may not fulfil the criteria for true protocol biopsies. It is important in order to achieve high diagnostic yield from transbronchial biopsies and cytology to have histopathologists trained in the specialized area of lung transplantation pathology and to maintain a close clinical liaison with the respiratory transplant physician and microbiologist in particular. There are however some clinical situations where non-invasive investigations suggest lung pathology but bronchoscopy with biopsy and cytology have failed to establish a diagnosis. Under these circumstances an open lung biopsy through video-assisted thoracoscopy or a thoracotomy may be considered. Occasionally a lung transplant recipient will undergo acute deterioration where a definitive diagnosis on transbronchial biopsy is considered unlikely and risky and a decision is therefore made to proceed to a single invasive procedure. In the acute situation empirical treatment may have been commenced despite the absence of a specific diagnosis and indeed to cover more than one diagnostic possibility. The interpretation of pathologic changes in open lung biopsies must therefore be made with care when recent treatment may have modified the histologic appearances.

Results from a number of centers have shown that despite the increased amount of tissue available in an open biopsy a new diagnosis as compared with the preceding transbronchial biopsy is only made in approximately 30% of cases with confirmation of a previous diagnosis in a similar number. The yield of new diagnoses is greater in longer survivors and there seems to be little benefit from the procedure within the first 6 weeks post-transplantation. Open lung biopsy diagnoses made in the early transplant period are often of treatable conditions such as infection whereas those made in the later postoperative period are most commonly chronic rejection, i.e. obliterative bronchiolitis, and bronchiolitis obliterans organizing pneumonia. The extra yield from open biopsy in the acute clinical situation is similar to other groups of immunocompromised patients, but in the lung transplant recipient the additional potential diagnosis of acute rejection as a sole or concomitant process may drive the requirement for an open biopsy sample. In addition to unsuspected infection, post-transplant lymphoproliferative disease may be diagnosed for the first time or confirmed on open lung biopsy. A previous suggestive transbronchial biopsy may not have yielded sufficient tissue or tumor to allow adequate histologic classification of its nature.

Open lung biopsy may also be of value where there is a suspicion of recurrence of primary disease in the graft, further widening the differential diagnosis. Less than 4% of patients in our program have required open lung biopsy. The majority of these were performed at a mean of 24 months following transplantation. All of these late biopsies showed changes of obliterative bronchiolitis of varying severity with changes of chronic vascular rejection and additional features of organizing pneumonia, fungal infection and recurrent disease in 40% of the cases. The open lung biopsies performed within the first 6 months following transplantation showed diffuse alveolar damage with CMV pneumonitis, acute rejection and necrotizing bronchiolitis respectively and two of these patients died within one week of the biopsy. The working formulation for the classification of lung rejection can be applied in practice in open lung biopsy material although it is strictly based on transbronchial biopsy specimens. It should however be applied with this caveat in mind.

A selection of diagnoses made on open lung biopsy are illustrated in this section.

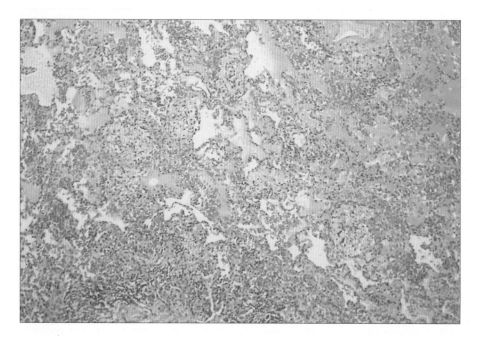

Figure 37.1
An open biopsy performed in the first 6 months following transplantation for undiagnosed clinical deterioration shows pneumonic consolidation with inflammation, hemorrhage and edema. No perivascular distribution to the infiltration is seen.

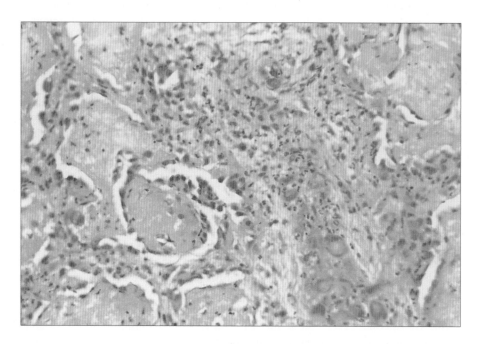

Figure 37.2
Higher power shows numerous cytomegalovirus (CMV) infected cells with polymorphs infiltrating and forming collections together with fibrin and type 2 pneumocyte hyperplasia. This confirms the diagnosis to be CMV pneumonitis. The patient continued to deteriorate despite CMV treatment and died with disseminated CMV disease.

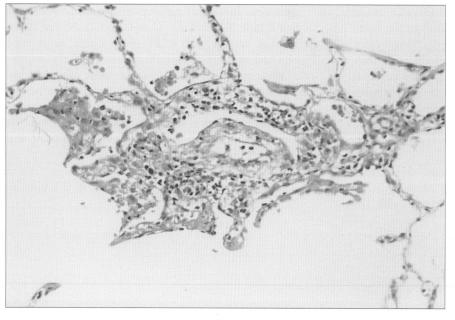

Figure 37.3
An open lung biopsy showed a single perivascular infiltrate with some polymorphs and intra-alveolar macrophages. Grading this infiltrate is not strictly possible due to the other features strongly suggestive of infection and it is unlikely that with this *single* perivascular lesion the unexplained clinical deterioration was all due to acute pulmonary rejection.

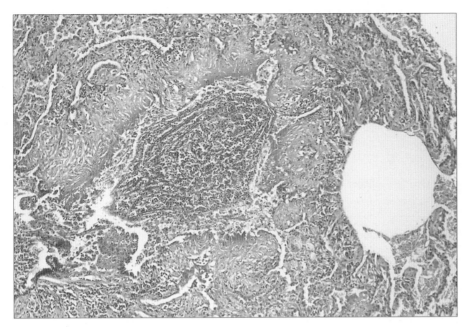

Figure 37.4
Another open lung biopsy which shows a necrotizing bronchiolitis which was present diffusely throughout the sample. No organism was cultured nor was there evidence of opportunistic infection histologically. The patient had been transplanted for bronchiectasis of unknown cause raising the possibility that this diffuse bronchiolitis could represent recurrence of a preoperative condition. It must be noted however that all patients with obliterative bronchiolitis develop bronchiectasis as part of their chronic airways rejection and so the true incidence of recurrence of any form of bronchiectasis with small airways disease cannot be adequately assessed in this group of patients.

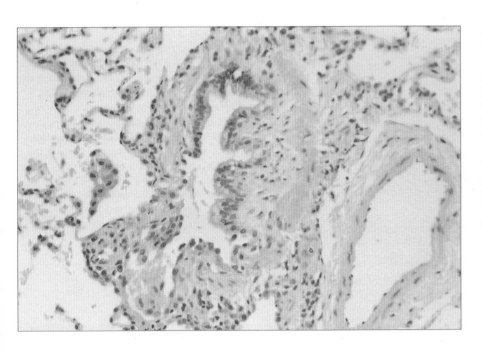

Figure 37.5
Open biopsy taken in the late post-transplant period showing a bronchiole with a mild peribronchiolar inflammatory infiltrate and an increase in loose fibrous tissue between the epithelium and the muscularis. The abnormal fibrous tissue encroaches on the lumen. The respiratory epithelium is intact for approximately half of the bronchiolar surface and attenuated and flattened for the remainder. The accompanying vessel appears unremarkable. This patient had not shown evidence of obliterative bronchiolitis on previous transbronchial biopsies. Obliterative bronchiolitis is diagnosed on this occasion.

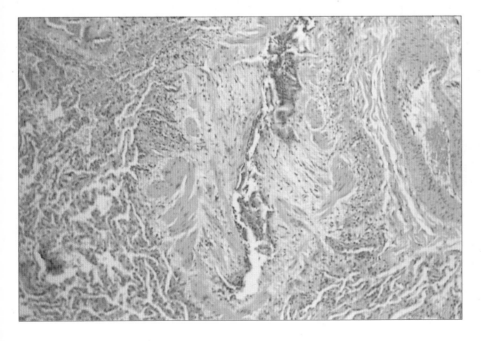

Figure 37.6
A further open lung biopsy showing much more advanced obliterative bronchiolitis with almost complete occlusion of the lumen by loose fibrous tissue which has breached and destroyed part of the muscle coat. There is background inflammation in the parenchyma predominantly of interstitial nature but no significant lymphocytic infiltrate associated with the fibrosis. The remaining epithelium appears in places to be hyperplastic.

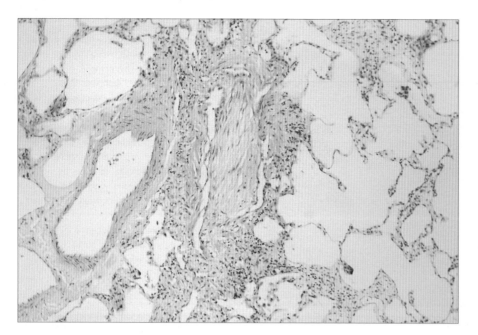

Figure 37.7

Open lung biopsy showing a bronchiole along side an unremarkable artery. The lumen of the bronchiole is almost entirely obliterated by loose fibrous tissue associated with a mild inflammatory infiltrate at its periphery. This represents involvement of a distal bronchiole by organizing pneumonia rather than obliterative bronchiolitis. This distinction is more easily made on an open biopsy than transbronchial biopsy.

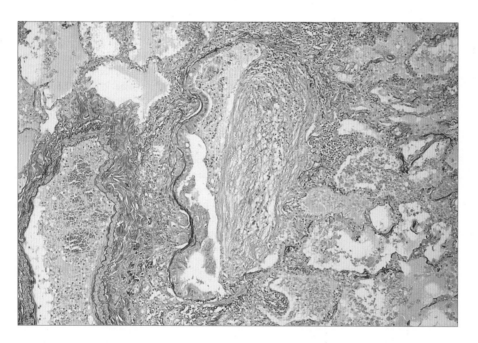

Figure 37.8

Connective tissue stain shows an eccentric fibrous plaque with loose fibromyxoid tissue and foamy macrophages and destruction of the elastica of the bronchiolar wall. The lesion is unusual for its eccentric location but is otherwise entirely consistent with obliterative bronchiolitis. In unusual cases such as this it is important to exclude the lesion being part of a bronchiolitis obliterans organizing pneumonia by examining all the material including deeper levels. No such lesion was present in this case, and the diagnosis of obliterative bronchiolitis was offered.

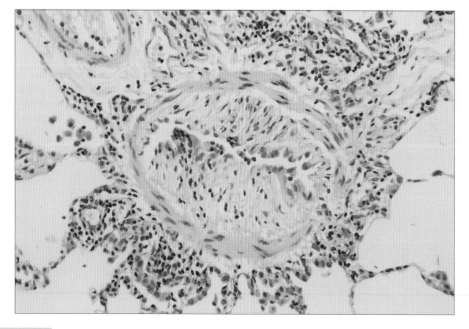

Figure 37.9

Open lung biopsy showing obliterative bronchiolitis with almost total reduction in the lumen with preservation of the smooth muscle and cuboidal metaplasia of the epithelium. There is quite an intense peribronchiolar infiltrate which may imply that augmented immunosuppression may prevent or halt the progression of lesions elsewhere in the lung. It is unlikely that further enhanced immunosuppression will reverse established acellular fibrosis in heavily scarred airways.

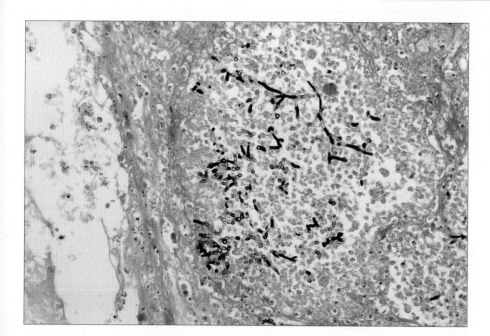

Figure 37.10
Open lung biopsy showing a necrotizing area with fungus present on silver staining. Other fields of the biopsy showed established obliterative bronchiolitis. This fungus has appearances consistent with *Aspergillus*, but in addition *Petrillydium boydii* was cultured.

FURTHER READING

Chaparro C, Maurer JR, Chamberlain DW, Todd TR. Role of open lung biopsy for diagnosis in lung transplant recipients: Ten-year experience. *Ann Thorac Surg* 1995;59:928–32.

APPENDIX 1

Rapid biopsy processing

Program title: Two-hour process
Program number: 2

Position	Reagent	Conc (%)	Temp	Vac	Drain	Time
1	NBF	10	37	Y	1:15	00.22
2	Alcoholic formalin		38	Y	1:15	00.10
3	Alcohol	90	39	Y	1:15	00.03
4	Alcohol 1	74 OP	40	Y	1:15	00.05
5	Alcohol 2	74 OP	40	Y	1:15	00.05
6	Alcohol 3	74 OP	40	Y	1:15	00.05
7	Alcohol/Xylene	50 / 50	40	Y	1:45	00.04
8	Xylene 1		41	Y	1:30	00.05
9	Xylene 2		43	Y	1:30	00.05
10	Xylene 3		45	Y	1:30	00.08
11	Wax 1		60	Y	1:45	00.12
12	Wax 2		60	Y	1:50	00.15

Processing programs used on a Shandon Pathcentre™ enclosed tissue processor.

Histology staining method: Perls' elastic van Gieson

References:	Miller PJ. An elastin stain. *Med Lab Technol* 1971;**28**(2):148–9.
	Bancroft & Cook. *Manual of Histological Techniques*. 1984. Churchill Livingstone, London.

Control tissue: Lung containing hemosiderin

Sections: Routine paraffin following neutral buffered formalin fixation

Solutions:
A 0.3% potassium permanganate
B 1% oxalic acid
C Perls' reagent: 25 ml 2% aqueous hydrochloric acid
                            25 ml 2% potassium ferrocyanide
D Miller's stain
E Harris hematoxylin
F 1% Hydrochloric acid in 70% alcohol
G van Gieson

Method:
1 Sections to water
2 Oxidize in 0.3% potassium permanganate, 5 minutes
3 Wash in running tap water
4 Decolorize in 1% oxalic acid
5 Rinse in running tap water followed by distilled water
6 Perls' reagent 15 minutes
7 Wash in running tap water
8 Rinse in 70% alcohol
9 Stain in Miller's for 60 minutes
10 Rinse in 70% alcohol
11 Wash in running tap water
12 Stain in Harris Hematoxylin 5 minutes
13 Wash in running tap water
14 Differentiate in 1% acid alcohol for 10 seconds
15 Wash in running tap water
16 Counterstain in van Gieson for 3 minutes
17 Dehydrate *rapidly*, clear and mount

Results:

Elastin fibers	Black
Collagen	Red
Nuclei	Blue
Muscle/cytoplasm	Yellow
Ferric iron	Blue

Notes:
I   Washing in water after van Gieson should be avoided as the color balance will be impaired. BLOT dry followed by industrial methylated spirits.
II   See Control of Substances Hazards to Health (COSHH) data sheets for chemicals used in method.
III Nuclear staining should be intense before van Gieson application as the picric acid will act as a differentiator.
IV **Picric acid is *explosive* when dry.**

APPENDIX 3

Histology staining method: Masson trichrome

Reference: Masson P (1929) Some histological methods. Trichrome stainings and their preliminary technique. *Bull Internat Ass Med*;**12**:75.

Control tissue: Muscle fibers

Sections: Routine paraffin wax following formalin fixation

Solutions:
    A Weigert's hematoxylin
    B 1% Hydrochloric acid in 70% alcohol
    C Masson red
       0.5% Ponceau 2R in 1% acetic acid 50 ml
       0.5% Acid fuchsin in 1% acetic acid 50 ml
    D 2% Aqueous phosphomolybdic acid
    E Masson green
       0.2% light green in 0.2% acetic acid

Method:
1. Take sections to water
2. Weigert's hematoxylin 10 minutes
3. Running tap water
4. Differentiate in acid alcohol 10–15 seconds
5. Running tap water
6. Masson red 5 minutes
7. Wash in running tap water
8. Phosphomolybdic acid 1 minute
9. Drain slides, then treat with Masson green 1 minute
10. Wash in distilled water
11. Dehydrate, clear and mount

Results:
Cytoplasm, muscle, red blood cells	– Red
Basement membranes, collagen	– Green
Nuclei	– Blue/Black

Notes:
    I   See COSHH data sheets for chemicals used in the method
    II Differentiation with phosphomolybdic acid is critical. It should be carried out until the connective tissue is almost unstained.
    III Ponceau 2R is also known as Ponceau de xylidine.

Histology staining method: rapid Grocott

Introduction: This technique is used to demostrate the presence of fungus and/or *Pneumocystis carinii*. The chromic acid oxidises the carbohydrate coat of the fungi to aldehydes which reduce the hexamine silver nitrate to a black metallic sliver compound.

Reference: Grocott RG (1955) *Am J Pathol*;**25**:975.

Control tissue: Tissue containing fungi and *P. carinii*

Sections: Routine paraffin following neutral buffered formalin fixation

Solutions:
- A   5% Chromic acid (chromium trioxide solution)
- B   1% aqueous sodium metabisulphite
- C   Stock hexamine silver solution: (store at 4°C)
  - 5% Silver nitrate 10 ml
  - 3% Hexamine 200 ml
- D   Working silver solution:
  - Stock   25 ml
  - Borax   4 ml
  - Distilled water   25 ml
- E   0.02% Gold chloride
- F   5% Sodium thiosulphate
- G   1% aqueous light green

Method:
1. Place chromic acid in 56°C water bath
2. Make up silver solution and place in same water bath at least 10 minutes before starting the method.
3. Sections to water
4. 5% Chromic acid at 56°C for 8 minutes
5. Rinse in running tap water
6. Sodium metabisulphite for 1 minute
7. Wash well in running tap water
8. Rinse in several changes of distilled water
9. Place in heated silver solution and check microscopically after 15 minutes. (The maximum time should be 20 minutes if silver is up to temperature).
10. Rinse in several changes of distilled water
11. Tone in gold chloride 30 seconds
12. Rinse in distilled water
13. Fix in sodium thiosulphate for 5 minutes
14. Wash well in running tap water
15. Wash in distilled water
16. Counterstain with light green for 30 seconds
17. Rinse in tap water
18. Dehydrate, clear and mount

Results:

Fungal hyphae walls and *P carinii*	– Black
Mucus, melanin and glycogen	– Grey
Background	– Light Green

COSHH:
- I   *Chromic acid* – This substance causes severe burns and sensitization by skin contact. Always wear gloves when handling. In powder form the material is combustible.
- II   *Sodium metabisulphate* – Contact with acids liberates toxic fumes. Contact with eyes may cause severe damage. Always handle over ventilated surface wearing gloves and eye protection.

III *Hexamine* – May cause sensitization, wear gloves when handling.

IV *Silver nitrate* – This substance is midly corrosive, wear gloves when handling.

V *Gold chloride* – Is harmful if in contact with skin, eyes, nose and throat. Always use in ventilated area wearing gloves and eye protection.

VI *Light green* – Stain in powder form can cause respiratory irritation. Always weigh out in fume cupboard.

VII *Working silver solution* – If this solution is allowed to percipitate it may become expolsive. De-activate silver solution with 2% hydrochloric acid.

VIII For specific information on these substances consult the COSHH file.

Notes: i   Silver solution must be kept at 56°C before use

ii   Over oxidation in chromic acid will cause silver deposition on collagen.

Papworth transplant unit database: endomyocardial biopsy grading of cardiac rejection

A. **Patient data** Surname: Forename:

B. **Lab data** Transplant no: Lab no: Date of biopsy:

C. **Histopathologic assessment:**
1. **Grading of rejection**
(i) Rejection grade: . . . . □
    (Non-gradeable = 9)
(ii) Biopsy material: . . . . □
   • adequate for assessment = 1
   • insufficient = 2
   • inappropriate = 3
2. **Infective process**
(i) Histology suspicious of infection (No = 0, Yes = 1) . . . . □
(ii) Histologic process: . . . . □
   • invasive = 1
   • colonization = 2
(iii) Organisms code (Not identified 0) . . . . □

3. **Additional information**
(i) Previous biopsy site reaction present (No = 0, Yes = 1) . . . . □
(ii) Endocardial infiltrates present . . . . □
   • none = 0
   • with myocyte encroachment = 1
   • without myocardial encroachment = 2
(iii) Other lymphoproliferative present (No = 0, Yes = 1). . . . . □
(iv) Conspicuous fibrosis:. . . . . □
   • absent = 1
   • predom. interstitial = 1
   • predom. endocardial = 2
   • endocard./interstitial = 3
(v) Other abnormality present (No = 0, Yes, non-spec = 1). . . . . □
Specify:
   • peritransplant injury = 2
   • myocard. vascular change (A-sclerosis) = 3
   • epicard. vascular change (A-sclerosis) = 4
   • epicard. inflammation = 5
   • epicard. lipogranulomata = 6
   • myocard. calcification = 7
   • resolving/resolved rejection = 8
   • ischemic/infarct damage = 9

Comment:

APPENDIX 6

Papworth transplant unit database: transbronchial biopsy grading of pulmonary rejection

A. **Patient data** Surname: Forename:

B. **Lab data** Transplant no: Lab no: Date of biopsy:

C. **Grading of rejection**
(i)   Rejection grade: . . . . □
      (Non-gradeable = 9)
(ii) Biopsy material: . . . . □
      • adequate for assessment = 1
      • insufficient = 2
      • inappropriate = 3

2. **Infective process**
(i)   Histology suspicious of infection (No = 0, Yes = 1). . . . . □
(ii) Organism code:. . . . . □
      (Not identified = 0)
(iii) CMV . . . . □
      • infection = 1
      • Pneumonitis = 2
(iv) *Aspergillus* . . . . □
      • Tracheobronchial;   Invasive = 1
                             Saprophytic = 2
                             BCG = 3
      • Parenchymal;   Invasive – 4
                             Cavity = 5
      • Other = 6
        (specify..)

3. **Additional information**
(i)   Evidence of organizing pneumonia (No = 0, Yes = 1) . . . . □
(ii) Evidence of EBV-related (No = 0, Yes = 1) . . . . □
      Lymphoproliferative disorder
(iii) Other abnormality present (No = 0, Yes, Non-specific = 1). . . . . □
      Specify:
      • prominent bronchial assoc lymphoid tissue = 2
      • previous biopsy site = 3
      • evidence of aspiration = 4
      • evidence of resolved/resolving rejection = 5
      • hemorrhagic infarction = 6
      • recurrence of primary disease = 7
      • granulomatous inflammation = 8
      • diffuse alveolar damage = 9

INDEX

Note: Page references in **bold** refer to photographs